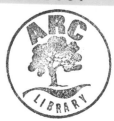
This book is dedicated to color vision deficient people and carriers of the factor—both in my family and elsewhere.

Many thanks to all the fine people who helped with finding the sources needed to compile this information.

COLOR VISION DEFICIENCY

and

COLOR BLINDNESS

An Introduction to the Problem

by

Mary Margaret Olsen
and
Kenneth R. Harris

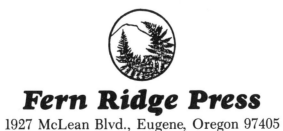

Fern Ridge Press

1927 McLean Blvd., Eugene, Oregon 97405

COLOR VISION DEFICIENCY AND COLOR BLINDNESS
An Introduction to the Problem

ISBN 0-9615332-2-6 (softbound)
SAN 695-0868

Fern Ridge Press
1927 McLean Blvd.
Eugene, OR 97405

Text input by:
Harris Educational Consultants
1408 Lawrence St.
Eugene, OR 97401

Digital phototype by
Editing & Design Services
30 East 13th Avenue
Eugene, OR 97401

TABLE OF CONTENTS

Color Vision Deficiency...1

Adult Problems..3

Problems of Children..9

Hereditary and Non-Hereditary Factors Causing
    Color Vision Deficiency.. 17

Tests for Color Vision..23

What Do the Color Deficient See? 29

How We See.. 31

Treatment...35

Bibliography..39

Supplemental Reading... 45

Index...53

Glossary..59

Color Vision Deficiency

The term "color blind" is usually a misnomer. While it is true that there are a few people who cannot see any color (they see life as in a black and white movie), they only comprise about 0.003 percent of the male population. (Burnham, Hanes and Bartleson) Most people with color vision problems do see some color. A better term is "color deficient" and will be used hereafter. The general public is more familiar with the term "color blind," and many research materials are listed under that designation.

Because there are at least seven color deficient males to every one color deficient female in the United States, he, his and him are used in this material in referring to the color deficient. Color deficient females, though rarer, have all of the same problems as the males, and have an equal right to consideration.

Generally speaking, people are not aware that there are possible employment problems and potential difficulties in school for color deficient persons.

Few articles have been published on color vision deficiency (color blindness) in periodicals for lay people, and those few, brief and superficial. While there is information on the subject in professional journals, the average person will not find the material readily available nor easily readable. There has never been a readily available, extensive listing, or explanation of employment and education problems affecting people with color vision deficiency.

The material has not been available to those who need it most, the affected, their families and teachers. This is an attempt to bring together some of the material on the subject in the hope that it will provide some useful insight into the problems faced everyday by those suffering from color deficiency.

Adult Problems

Color deficiency is poorly understood by most people. Since it is not deadly, painful, disfiguring nor socially ostracising, it is usually regarded as an unimportant physical factor by the majority of both professionals and lay persons.

In *The Handicap of Color Blindness*, Dr. Heath writes, "Regretably, it is probably not very unfair to say that the overwhelming majority of optometrists or other vision care experts today could not . . . even describe the main handicaps or shortcomings in everyday activities that might result from a particular defect in color perception."

Ultimately, it is in the vocational world that the color deficient individual may find his gravest problems. During the high school years, wisely pkanned vocational decisions are important. Many students go no farther than high school, and need to make the most of all available education while there. For those going on to college, the ground work for many careers can be improved by adequate course choices in high school. Certainly, a student needs to know about his color vision before he puts time and money into higher education. The use of color coding has increased greatly in the past few decades. All young people should be screened for color vision perception before they choose a career. A color deficient student may find that putting a great deal of time into electronics may not be productive. He may decide it would be wiser not to plan on going into law enforcement, interior decorating, etc.

One year, recently, I contacted the counselors at five local high schools. None of them were aware that, statistically, four out of every hundred of their students was color deficient. None had ever received any information as to the possible problems faced by the color deficient person in the working world.

Indeed, the most important problems are faced in the working world. For some persons who are less seriously color deficient, this statement will be viewed with absolute disbelief. Many color deficient people who have been fortunate enough to become lawyers, accountants, educators, business managers, architects, actors, musicians, singers, etc. may have seldom or never had problems because of color deficiency. They often find it difficult to believe that color deficiency can be a severe hindrance.

Many researchers have commented on the fact that some color deficient persons are not aware of their problem. Failure to pass a color vision test may be their first encounter with the information, and they often cannot accept the fact. (Pickford, 1951) They think the tests are wrong, or the person testing made a mistake because many color deficient persons have had no problems in daily life. (Heath, 1974)

R.W. Pickford (1951) states that it may be difficult to understand that a man who cannot distinguish red from green should think that he has normal color vision, but he has never seen the difference between these colors as the average person sees them, and there is no way of enabling him to do so.

Eight out of every hundred males in the U.S. are color deficient, and about .06 percent of females. Of the color deficient people, the anomalous trichromat is the least color deficient. Three out of four color deficient persons fall into this category. They confuse reds and greens with browns. Dichromats have a more severe problem. They confuse reds, greens and browns with grays. Some dichromats see red as black. Many color deficient persons see purple as blue.

The anomalous trichromat is the most likely to be unaware of his deficiency. The dichromat usually does know because his problem is more severe, and he has had color vision difficulties of various kinds most of his life. (Heath, 1974)

It would save people time, expense, and disappointment if all color deficient people could know of their complications before any problems occur. Dr. Cruz-Coke says that color deficiency ". . . disqualifies a man from several occupations in a society which uses color as signals in traffic lights, on labels, railroads, planes, art and industry. Testing for color blindness should, therefore, be included in the physical examination of school children and the results utilized for vocational counseling."

In the U.S. Armed Services, the Army will accept more color deficient persons than will the Navy or Air Force. In all the Services, there are many areas of work which are closed to the color deficient. (Personal interviews, U.S. Armed Services, 1987)

The United States Dept. of Transportation requires a color vision test for some drivers in interstate commerce, (Fed. Highway Admin. Regulations, 1980), and for water pilots, "No license as master, mate, or pilot of any class of vessel shall be renewed without furnishing a satisfactory certificate of examination as to color blindness." (U.S.Code, 1976 Ed.,v.ll,Title 46)

Even though one might hesitate to recommend art as a vocation for a young color deficient person, people have actually succeeded as artists. The color deficient person might combine his colors in unexpected ways, but this might render his art more intertesting.

Pickford (1964) tells of a young man who made his living as a portrait and landscape artist even though he was deuteranomalous (green-weak). Some famous painters who have been suspected of being color deficient include Whistler, Carriers, and Grottger. The artist Leger was actually proved to be color deficient. Dr. Snyder, himself color deficient, is an artist, among other things, and he uses colors in his paintings.

Researchers have found that the color deficient person is often very uncomfortable about his problem. While most other vision abnormalities do not make people feel this way, the color deficient person is likely to be defensive about his color deficiency. He does not want it discussed. (Peters)

In their childhoods, many color deficient persons have suffered from teasing and ridicule. Efforts should be made to avoid allowing this kind of thing to happen to these children.

Color deficient adults will seldom ask for help with their color problems. My color deficient sister loved to sew, but she often had trouble matching her thread to her material. She would never explain the situation to a clerk and ask for help, though they would have been glad to help her. One writer states that he often rented cars in his work, but had trouble finding them after parking. A policeman once even became suspicious of this man when he had trouble locating his car but the man did not try to explain. That he did not want to explain is typical of most color deficient people. (Davids)

The following is only a partial list of employment areas which either may, or probably will, present problems for the color deficient person:

Electronics	Florist
Fashion design	Dyeing industry
Pilot, air or water	Some truck driving
Interior decorating	Geologist
Chemist	Wallpaper hanger
Biologist	Dressmaker
Printer	Weaver
Upholsterer	Tailor
Some work with computers	Many positions, U.S.
House Painting	Armed Services

Many color deficient people have told me that their greatest annoyance with colors is with their clothing. Not all color deficient persons have a wife, mother, sister, or other helpful relative around to help them with their clothes. Some suggestions that might prove useful are, purchase some medium sized safety pins and pin a pair of socks together before putting them in the wash. Leave them pinned together until you wear them. Johnson (as an adult) solved the problem of matching his socks by wearing boots. Very clever! Boots are now made to wear with almost anything.

When purchasing clothes, you can tell which ones are black, white or shades of gray. You can almost certainly distinguish the yellows and probably blues. Tell the clerk that you are partially color blind and that you don't want clothing in any shades of green, red, orange or purple, (or pink) at all. If a clerk does not seem cooperative, ask to see the manager and explain your situation.

You can purchase a pen for marking your clothes (from a dry cleaners if you can't find one elsewhere). Some people number their clothes, devising a numbering system so they know what they want to wear with which clothes. If you receive clothes for presents, ask the giver what color it is if you aren't sure. If they say something like mauve or taupe or magenta, or some other word that is meaningless to you, ask if that is a shade of red or brown or whatever.

Most wives are very helpful to their husbands in dealing with their clothes. However, a few are not. I once met a professional woman who stated that her color deficient husband always wanted her to go with him when he bought clothes. She said, "He really doesn't need help, he just wants attention". Well, he wasn't just asking for attention, and in my opinion, she must be a woman of little imagination or empathy to feel that way.

If a family wants their color deficient relative to enjoy their flower garden, plant some white, yellow and blue flowers, and use some plants with varigated foliage (and even gray tones, like Dusty Miller). Green plants with red or orange flowers just look shades of brown to most color deficient people.

I could make the same suggestion about colors for interior decorating. Since reds, greens, and maybe oranges will appear in shades of brown, one could end up with a very brown room as far as the color deficient person is concerned. And purple (and pink!) may be seen as blue. Use contrasts, light colors against dark colors, etc.

I have noticed that most color deficient people seem to like brown. Understandable . . . their world may be full of it, and brown is a warm and comfortable color.

It is unfortunate that red and green were chosen for our traffic light. Before 1931, many drivers were having some trouble distinguishing the colors of traffic lights. In 1931, the International Commission on Illumination at Cambridge adopted some resolutions concerning traffic light colors. The Institute of Transportation Engineers has set standards based on these resolutions. The green lights tend to be in the blue-green zone and the red lights may have some orange overtones. (U.S.Dept. of Transportation, Federal Highway Admin.) After the changes instituted in 1931, most color deficient persons have found it easier to distinguish the traffic light colors. Also, the red is on top and the green on the bottom. Horizontaly, the red light is on the left.

I would like to make another suggestion to the families of color deficient people. Keep an eye on traffic lights, especially any place where new traffic lights are installed. The green lights are supposed to be colored toward the blue side, not the yellow. In my city, I see some new traffic lights as decidedly more yellow than the other green traffic lights in town. Anyone can send for a copy of the Vehicle Traffic Control Signal Heads, A Standard of the Institute of Transportation Engineers, from the Federal Highway Admin. (See bibliography). In this city, I think the city traffic engineer accepts whatever shade of green the supplier sends. I questioned one of our traffic engineers and he did not know anything about the color standards. That may be true in most cities. People can question their own city engineers. At the end of the bibliography is a list of some of the suppliers of traffic signal lights.

Originally, people wore red for hunting caps and vests. Some long time ago, the color was changed to orange though, as yet, not all states have adopted it. It is a much better choice, especially if 'neon' orange is used. However, I feel that bright yellow would be even better.

Two well known men of our own time who are or were color deficient are Bing Crosby and Paul Newman. The daughters of these men are all carriers of the factor. There have to be dozens more color deficient persons among the well known, but we just don't know who they are.

In his well researched, biographical novel of Mary Todd Lincoln, *Love is Eternal*, Irving Stone has Abraham Lincoln say that he never cared for flowers because he could not tell colors.

Color vision deficiency is poorly understood by most people and few could tell you of the possible problems facing the color deficient person. Each of us must attempt to put ourselves in the position of the color deficient, considering educational, occupational, and emotional effects of that condition.

Problems of Children

Parents need to be aware that in kindergarten and in the primary grades, color plays an extremely important part in the education and activities of children. For example, in the Functional Color Component (FCC) approach to reading instruction, Sassenroth, Pierce and Maddux found that it uses color codes to teach sounds, silent letters, vowels, etc. For example, consonant sounds are red and green, silent letters and short vowels are yellow, long vowels are usually orange. In all, five colors are used. There are other publishers using words in colored print to designate different things, as well as using colored pictures. (Sewell)

In her doctoral dissertation on color deficiency, Wildman tells us that some first grade reading readiness books contain directions using color and some arithmetic books require that the students match figures or symbols by color.

'Cuisenaire Rods' have been used extensively to teach arithmetic in kindergarten, first and second grades. The system teaches children numbers by measuring with colored wooden or plastic rods instead of using numerals. There are other similar arithmetic systems such as Stern's 'Structural Arithmetic', which uses colored blocks. (Sharp) 'Math Their Way' uses color cubes, colored pattern blocks, and there are many other colored items to use with it, such as colored beads, colored buttons, Unifix snap-together cubes, etc. (Personal observation by the author and items in Lakeshore Curriculum Materials catalog.) All of these are lovely and are probably pleasant and helpful for the average child, but present serious problems for the color deficient child.

You can imagine how the color deficient child must feel when presented with these materials and instructions to use them. Red and green are used in these materials. They would probably look shades of brown. If purple is used, it can be seen as blue by some color deficient children.

Many kinds of learning games are used through the elementary school years. Some are devised by teachers, and some are produced commercially. To play many of these games, recognition of colors is essential. Of course, some are designed to teach colors.

Some researchers have been able to test whole school or school district populations. They have found that for most of the affected students, neither the students, nor their parents or teachers were aware of their color deficiency. (Litton: Dvorine)

Dr. Thuline (1964) states that not only do these color deficient children have problems but they do not know the reason for the problems. Usually, their parents are just as unaware. But even if they do know their child is color deficient, parents tend to regard the fact as a curiosity, since they are not aware of the difficulties facing their child. Thuline reports that parents have said, "I'm glad to know what the problem is since we thought he must be dumb about learning his colors". About an older student, another said, "That explains his terrible taste in clothes."

When dealing with color deficient children, it is reasonable to assume that the attitudes of parents and the frustrations of teachers will have some effect on the child's behavior. (Thuline, 1964)

A kindergarten teacher said she was having considerable trouble with a little girl, especially at finger painting time. It was recommended that she be tested for color deficiency. The whole class was tested and the girl and two boys were found to be color deficient. All three children had presented occasional social problems, especially when colors were concerned. (Basford) A test for color deficiency was conducted in the 1960s for grades 1,2, and 3 in the City Schools of Murfreesboro, Tennessee. A total of 1,295 pupils were tested. In that test, thirty nine boys and two girls were found to be color deficient, but the pupils, parents and teachers were not aware of the defect. (Shearron, 1965)

In London, England, studies done in some primary and junior schools revealed that none of the teachers of the 8,755 children tested knew of any child's color deficiency. Nevertheless, an average amount of color deficiency (four out of 100 children) was found among the students. (Waddington)

Untrained people who deal with color deficient children may attribute the inability to distinguish colors to stupidity and become impatient with them when they are slow in answering. (Cobb; Espinda)

Obviously, the color deficient child who cannot perceive the colors he is required to use is likely to feel very frustrated, according to Dr. Heath. (1974) Researchers studying this problem have seen evidence of such emotional factors as anxiety, shame, and fear of ridicule in affected children. (Litton)

When a child becomes aware that he is different from others, he may react by withdrawing or by becoming difficult to manage. Color deficient children often exhibit one of these extremes. (Basford)

Dr. Snyder, a researcher who was himself color deficient, remembers that during the winter he colored the grass in his pictures brown. Later in the year, he continued to color it brown. (Grass probably looked brown to him all the time.) He had to memorize the fact that grass is green in the summer, where he lives. He had to memorize colors for fire engines, water, auto tires, oranges and many other things. Crayons have the color names printed on the paper wrappers. (If the wrappers are gone, the color deficient child is in trouble!)

Prof. Basford relates that, in the first grade, one little boy painted red leaves and green flowers on a bush. His teacher held it up to the class and said, "Look at this!" and everyone laughed. Because of this experience, the boy knew he was different, but he did not know why.

When writing about her color deficient son, Rosenberg says that her son showed a great lack of interest in colors. If he could help it, he didn't want to color anything but pumpkins because he knew which crayon to use for pumpkins. He chose the right crayon for coloring leaves green but only because he remembered the length of his green crayon. He would never touch jigsaw puzzles because working them depended upon recognizing color as much as upon recognizing shape.

It would be very helpful for the color deficient child if parents would print the color names on colored pencils, above the paints in water color paint boxes, and possibly, on some other things.

Julia Sewell developed a coding method for a color deficient student who was not yet reading. A red heart, yellow sun, purple grapes, brown basket, green tree, blue bird, black hat, orange orange symbols were used. The child memorized these symbols and the teacher put them in all the places where the child might need them.

Sewell also suggested that a color deficient child might ask another student to identify colors for him. This would not always succeed. A color deficient man told me that, when he was a child, his classmates would deliberately tell him the wrong colors when he asked them for help because they considered it laughable to do so.

So many games have colored pieces used for playing the games. With games in the home, parents could use acrylic paints and for red, green, orange, or purple pieces to be moved, paint the pieces in white, black, grey, yellow, blue, (with brown as a sixth choice). At least, your child could be more comfortable with games in the home.

Mary Waddington, lecturer in child development, tells us that color deficient children usually manage to hide their problems. Ridicule is difficult for children to cope with and those who have been laughed at for their color recognition mistakes will not willingly make those mistakes again. They learn to watch others, to copy others and to avoid situations involving color. They try very hard to conceal their problems.

Across the United States, most states do not test all school children for color deficiency. (Personal survey of all U.S. states, 1985) Some only give the test to learning disabled children.

It is unfortunate that attention is paid to color deficiency only when dealing with learning disabilities. Actually, color deficient children have not necessarily been found to be handicapped in their learning abilities. Evidence was provided in tests done in the Denver Public Schools in the first, second and third grades. Those tests focused on language, arithmetic, and social studies, and found no significant differences between color deficient pupils and those with average color vision. (Lampe, Doster & Beal)

The City Schools in Murfreesboro, Tenn. tested grades one, two and three for reading skills. No evidence was found of a relationship between color deficiency and reading achievement . (Shearron, 1964)

Dr. Anthony Adams says "Children who have difficulty distinguishing colors may be misdiagnosed as having learning difficulties unless the color vision defect is known."

Speaking of his own problems, Dr. Snyder found that learning about his own color deficiency was a relief because he hadn't known why he couldn't learn colors.

Many professionals in the fields of education and vision care believe that all children should be tested early for color vision deficiency.

Optometrist Joel Zaba believes that children should always be screened for color deficiency and parents and teachers should be informed if the child is color deficient because of the extensive use of color in early education.

Mary Waddington says, "It is important . . . that teachers should know as soon as possible if a child does not possess normal colour vision . . . ."

Dr. Snyder feels that, "An early diagnosis of color deficiency could lessen or eliminate the potentially frustrating and negative learning experiences of a color defective child."

The National Association of Vision Program Consultants states that, "Color vision tests are advised . . . and should given in Junior High or at least by grade 7, when vocational counseling usually begins.", and that lay volunteers, teachers, teacher aides, nurses, and/or specially trained personnel can all administer eye screening tests, but those without special training should receive a certain amount of advice or training in order to do the best at testing.

In its *"Vision Screening Guidelines for School Nurses"*, the National Association of School Nurses lists the following procedures on p.9,

Color Discrimination:

Screening for color discrimination is recommended because of educational or vocational implications. There is no treatment. Use the following procedure:

1. Use Ishihara or American Optical Test Books.
2. Instructions with the test should be followed.
3. Screen twice if first test is failed.
4. Test should be used with adequate daylight lighting.
5. Notify parent and teacher of test results.
6. Record results on permanent health record.

Even though color deficient children do not see all the colors, they should not be discouraged from enjoying artistic activities. There are many areas of artistic endeavor in which color is not necessarily important. Sculpture in clay, sculpture in stone, wood carving, metal working, leather working and making things with many kinds of natural materials can all be done without worrying about color. When it comes to drawing, it might help to notice just a few of the artists who are noted for their drawings. They are not color deficient but do many drawings which do not include color. Susan Perl has illustrated many appealing children's books with her line drawings of youngsters, as has Leonard Lublin.

Peter Parnall does wonderful line drawings of wild animals. Kit Dalton, Reina Rubel, Quentin Blake, Jean-Claude Suares, Karla Kuskin, Garth Williams, Wanda Gag and many, many more have illustrated children's books with fascinating line drawings.

Aubrey Beardsley and James Montgomery Flagg were both famous artists who did many line drawings. In Coos Bay, OR, Don R. Morrow does striking pencil drawings of beautiful old homes, along with other subjects.

And what about cartoonists? Those in the newspapers have earned income with line drawings.

One of my color deficient relatives began drawing as soon as he could hold a pencil. He loved to draw cars, trucks, planes, ships, etc. He drew for his own entertainment until he was about twelve and then stopped for his own reasons. When older, he did beautiful work with wood, wood marquetry, and leather. He has an unusually good sense of the contrasts of lights and darks and is a fine craftsman.

14

Another of my color deficient relatives builds beautiful scale models of historical subjects as a hobby and he not only exhibits them, but sometimes sells them.

Parents have been known to be very emotionally upset when they learn that their child is color deficient. People have said, "How sad that he cannot see all the beautiful colors." There is no need for anyone to feel this way. To begin with, he can see some color. In some ways, a color deficient child may 'see' more than the rest of his family. In his early developing years, the average person depends very much on his sense of color for identifying objects and learning about the world around him. The color deficient person learns early to rely on form, on design, on contrasts, on texture and on observation of motion to learn about his world. Actually, much of life's beauty and fascination has nothing to do with color. The shape of a leaf or the shape of a tree is every bit as beautiful as its color. Have you ever noticed? The way a seagull wheels down the sky is even more wonderful than its color.

Birds can be identified by their shapes, by their flight patterns, by the way they 'walk', and by their song as well as by the color of their feathers. We can miss a great deal in life if we rely chiefly on color in judging the world around us. Bees and some other insects see colors in the ultra-violet range which humans do not see. (Jonas and Jonas) Hummingbirds can also see near ultraviolet light. (Goldsmith) Do any people feel deprived because of that? We need to understand that the color deficient person finds the world as wonderful to see as anyone else. His world is just a little different.

There is a delightful little book entitled *Hailstones and Halibut Bones*, by Mary O'Neill which I wish all children could read. It is about colors, and has the most wonderful descriptions for each color, in poetry, through sound, sight, hearing, touch, smell, and feelings. For the color deficient child, it might give some idea of the colors they do not see, but for all children it will stretch the imagination and give much pleasure.

Everyone who is knowledgeable about color deficiency and children, and the world of employment feels that all school children should be tested for color vision during their school years.

I would like to see the time when all school children in the U.S. would be tested for color deficiency before they had to try to learn arithmetic or reading by colors, then see them tested again about seventh grade, and career counseling provided.

Working through the P.T.A. or other parent-teacher groups would be a good way to encourage color vision testing in schools. It might be wise for the parent-teacher group to go to the top (Superintendent or School Board) for permission before attempting to test their school. One parent-teacher group that I know of (a group of very good parents) decided they wanted to test the children in their school for color vision. They had permission from their principal and one school nurse said she would help. However, the head school nurse heard of it and said she didn't want it done, so the other school nurse could not help. The parents went ahead with it anyway, but it would have been very helpful for them to have had some trained help. Four different kinds of testing books were used, so all the children were not tested with the same materials. (I think that in testing other schools, all the children have been tested with the same kind of testing materials.) The people doing the testing were probably overly careful and found too many children whom they wanted re-tested. They had assumed at the beginning that the children they found would be re-tested. They never were re-tested so all the effort was for nothing.

If the parent-teacher group had gone either to the superintendent or the local school board first, I feel the results might have been different. I have reported this in order to help other groups of parents avoid problems.

If a parent-teacher group wanted to test a school or school district and materials were not available or not enough were available, it is possible that the local Lions Clubs or The Elks Lodge would purchase some materials for them for testing. Both groups give assistance with vision problems.

I would like to see the parents of color deficient children organize to see that the testing is done, and to see that color deficient children are not graded on color coded materials.

Parents groups might watch the traffic lights (see item in the chapter on Adult Problems) to see that yellow is not added to the green lights, that the lights are kept with a green shaded slightly toward blue, and a red shaded slightly toward orange.

They could collect information to apply toward career counseling and provide the information for high school counselors.

They might encourage manufacturers to use the colors yellow, black, white and gray as first choices whenever they were going to design any kind of color coding, with blue and brown added if they needed five or six colors.

Parents groups could develop creative ways to help color deficient persons with color coordinating their clothes, and develop printed materials for clothing store managers to use to alert their clerks that color deficient persons would appreciate a little sympathetic help.

Parents could unobtrusively observe their children, record problems and related occurences, and publish the results. Shirley Rosenberg, in her article, "The Boy Who Thought Pancakes Were Green," is the only parent I know of who has done so. However, please, do not make your child self-conscious about his color deficiency.

But first and most important, the children need to be tested for color vision.

Hereditary and Non-Hereditary Factors Causing Color Vision Deficiency

Many people who are aware of color deficiency know that it is hereditary but few have complete knowledge of all the factors involved.

If there were any color deficient people among your ancestors on either side, or among your living blood relations, you and your children should have your color vision tested by an optometrist, ophthalmogist, or family physician.

An article on genetic counseling says, "Some inherited disorders are transmitted by the mother and appear almost exclusively in their male children." These are known as X-linked recessive disorders, and include color blindness, hemophilia, and childhood muscular dystrophy, among others.

They are called X-linked recessive because they are carried on the X sex chromosome of the mother. (Willis)

Females have 2 X-chromosomes and males have one X and one Y-chromosome. A carrier (heterozygous) female has one normal X-chromosome and one X-chromosome with the color deficient factor. She can transmit the color deficient factor but is usually not color deficient herself. Each of her sons stands a 50 per cent chance of being color deficient and each of her daughters stands a 50 per cent chance of being a carrier of the factor. A color deficient (homozygous) female has to have two X-chromosomes with the color deficient factor. All of her sons will be color deficient and all of her daughters will be carriers. (Heath,1963; X-Chrom Manual)

Color deficient males do not transmit the factor to their children, as a rule, but all of their daughters will be carriers. (Genetic Counseling, March of Dimes Birth Defects Foundation) This is because the male children receive only a Y-chromosome from their fathers and the trait is carried on the X-chromosome, which they transmit to their daughters. Since the children of the color deficient male do not usually show the factor, many families mistakenly believe that the future family tree is free of the problem. Chart 1 shows the five possible ways for the inheritance of color deficiency to occur. Through the females, it is possible for the color deficient factor to go 'underground', so to speak, and subsequently to be passed on without any color deficient males appearing

18

for several generations. This possibility is greater in families with fewer children. (See Chart 2 at the end of this chapter.)

It may be that many genetic professionals, vision and medical doctors are not aware of the fact that a carrier {heterozygous} female can be somewhat color deficient herself. (Thuline, 1964 ; Volpe,) Some researchers feel that if all carrier females and other female relatives of the color deficient could be tested with the anomaloscope, many would prove to be color deficient to at least some degree. (Walls,Mathews; Kalmus)

Recent developments in genetics suggest that, although their color vision is relatively normal, some females who are heterozygous for the color vision deficient factor have eyes whose retinas must contain more than the usual three types of cones. Presumably, their retinas contain the three normal cone pigments and also an anomalous pigment because of the abnormal gene that they carry. (Nagy, MacLeod, Heyneman, & Eisner)

A geneticist once told me that, because my sister was color deficient, it meant that our mother was a carrier and our father was color deficient. Our father had passed away by that time, but we had never noticed any indication of color deficiency. We knew our mother was a carrier since one of her three sons was color deficient. Even if it had been true that our father was color deficient, all of his daughters would not necessarily have been homozygous for the color deficient factor. (Kalmus) (See No. 2, Chart 1) Statistically, half would have been homozygous for the factor and half heterozygous carriers of the factor. My sister's only son is not color deficient, but he would be if she had been homozygous for the factor. She was simply a heterozygous carrier who also exhibited the color deficient trait.

Dr. Horace Thuline (1964) writes, "The understandable reluctance physicians may have felt during the past in dealing with the parents of a color-vision defective girl, when the father was not affected, need no longer be a deterent to identifying such individuals".

Dr. Anthony Adams uses this chart,

HEREDITARY COLOR VISION DEFICIENCY INCIDENCE

Trichromats	Percentage in the male population
1. Normal	92.0
2. Deuteranomalous	5.0
3. Protanomalous	1.0
4. Tritanomalous	0.0001

Dichromats	
1. Deuteranopes	1.0
2. Protanopes	1.0
3. Tritanopes	0.001

Authors Deane B. Judd and Gunter Wyszechi (1963) write that, "In order to account for enough mothers for this eight per cent of red-confusing sons....., it follows that about sixteen per cent of all mothers are carriers." Only about 0.6 per cent of females are actually color deficient. (U.S. Dept. of Health, Ed. and Welfare) Color deficiency is found most frequently among peoples of European descent, but it occurs in all races. (Cruz-Coke)

There are many non-hereditary factors which may cause color deficiency. In the Journal of the American Optometric Association, (Jan.& Feb.,1974) Dr. Lyle wrote an extensive article on the drugs, chemicals, diseases and physical conditions which may alter color perception. This alteration is sometimes temporary and sometimes permanent. Lyle lists some 150 drugs and chemicals and some 70 diseases and other phytsical conditions which are associated with color deficiency.

Just a few of the drugs and chemicals listed are corticosteroids, digitalis, tobacco, alcohol and some industrial chemicals. A few of the diseases and physical conditions are multiple sclerosis, cataracts, glaucoma, diabetes, syphilis, pernicious anemia, some retinal vascular conditions, some injuries and deficiencies in vitamins A and D. Lyle states that,"It has been estimated that at least five per cent of the population have an aquired defect of color vision . . . ." Diabetics might do well to read the article by Shute and Oshinskie on possible color vision changes due to diabetes and self monitoring of blood sugar.

Researchers have noticed that yellow-blue vision tends to deteriorate somewhat in persons past middle age due to thickening of the lens of the eye. The thicker lens results in less light striking the retina, and since light is necessary for vision, the acuity and color sense of older adults are not as good as those of younger people. (Freese)

Any person noticing a change in his or her color vision should report the fact to his physician. Changes in color perception may be an early warning of a physical problem. (Adams)

Not long ago, I read in the newspaper that some families in Japan had made an interesting decision concerning the X-linked hereditary problems in their family lines. While these problems are passed on in family lines by both sexes, females usually only carry them on and do not exhibit them. The Japanese families had decided to try to have only female chilren so that they would have no children exhibiting the problems. A far better and permanent solution would be for the color deficient male to father only sons, since the trait is sex linked to the X-chromosome. This would remove it from the family line.

There are 205 confirmed or suspected catalogued disorders transmitted by a gene or genes on the X-chromosome. (Genetic Counseling, March of Dimes) With some of the serious disorders, I can certainly understand the decision those Japanese families made. While color vision deficiency is not a tragic disorder, some families might want to see if they could remove it from the family line, anyway.

I would like to mention another possible course, in case any family might wish to consider it. If a color deficient male fathered only sons, the deficiency factor would be out of his family as far as his own descendants were concerned.

Methods are being developed by which a couple may choose the sex of their offspring. At this time, I think that none of them are guaranteed.

The March of Dimes has a pamphlet, Genetic Counseling, and an International Directory of Genetic Services. Many cities across the U.S. have a March of Dimes office and it can be found in the phone book. For those places without such an office, you may contact:

March of Dimes Birth Defects Foundation
1275 Mamaroneck Ave.
White Planes, N.Y. 10605

Many states have teaching hospitals or health research centers from which current genetic research information may be obtained. Most of these places are listed in the March of Dimes material.

Color vision deficiency is a sex linked trait. Nationally, about eight percent of males in the U.S. are color deficient and about one half of one percent of the females are, also. Others, because of disease or chemical exposure, display color deficient symptoms but cannot transmit the acquired deficiency. The many drugs, chemicals and physical problems which can cause temporary or permanent color deficiency do not alter the genetic structure.

Only through heredity is color deficiency transmitted from generation to generation. The more we know of heredity the more we will know about those genetically transmitted traits such as color vision defidiency. It might behoove us all to learn more about heredity.

21

Chart 1
Hereditary Chart of Congenital Color Vision Deficiency

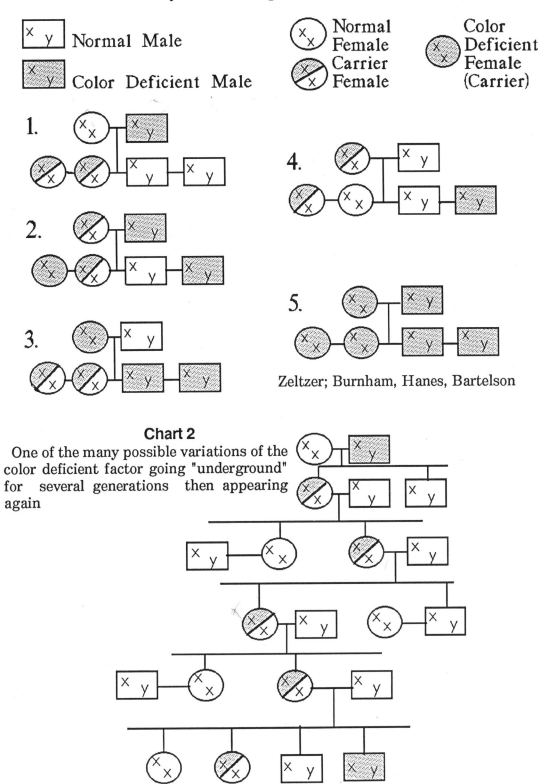

Zeltzer; Burnham, Hanes, Bartelson

Chart 2

One of the many possible variations of the color deficient factor going "underground" for several generations then appearing again

Tests for Color Vision

In an earlier chapter, the importance of testing all school age children for color vision deficiency was mentioned. Adults who feel that there is a possibility that they may have color deficient vision are also advised to seek color vision testing. These tests can be obtained through an optometrist, ophthalmologist, or one's family doctor.

Except for people who work with photography or with lighting, most people think of color mixtures of light in the same manner that they might think of color mixtures of pigments. But, actually, when a painter mixes pigments, the results differ from what happens when colors of light are mixed.

Red, blue and green are the primary colors of light and when the three primaries are added together, they create white light. Red and green lights added together yield yellow light. (Edge)

For many centuries, researchers have been interested in the way the eye perceives color. Various kinds of tests for measuring human color discrimination have been developed over the years.

The most complete and accurate tests for color vision are done using an anomaloscope, and two of the best known ones are the Rayleigh and Nagel anomaloscopes. Anomaloscopes are instruments which test color vision by having the subject look through an instrument with red, green and yellow filters. Light is shone through the filters. With the Nagel anomaloscope, the lower half is yellow, which can be made lighter or darker as the subject wishes when taking the test. The subject mixes red and green lights to match yellow light. Not only are these machines the most accurate, but they detect all types of color deficiency. There are many types of these machines, some using prisms and some using filters. Anomaloscopes are generally more expensive than some of the other testing devices, their use requires training, and most professionals do not have them. When using an anomaloscope, the average person makes a standard match when mixing red and green to match yellow, but the color deficient person makes other matches. (Renaldo) The terminology for classifying color vision deficient persons is taken from the results of testing done with anomaloscopes.

Persons with average color vision are classed as trichromnats. They can match all colors with mixtures of three colors. The largest group of color deficient persons can also do this, but their color matches are different. These people are classed as anomalous trichromats and their color deficiency is comparatively mild. These people are usually classed as 'red weak' (protanomalous) or as 'green weak' (deuteranomalous). More than half of all color deficient people are in these categories with deuteranomalous persons being the most common of the two. Persons classed as dichromats need only two colors to match all of the colors they see with the anomaloscope, and thus, their color deficiency is more severe. (They are aware that they have a problem). The two most common forms of dichromatic color deficiency are 'red blind' (protanopia) and 'green blind' (deuteranopia). (American Optometric Assoc. pamphlet)) People in all of these categories will have trouble with both reds and greens. (Heath, 1963)

A much less common form of color deficiency is yellow-blue deficiency (tritanomnalous and tritanopia). People with this form will not have as many employment problems as those with red-green deficiency, but many of the factors involved in both employment and social life would also apply to them. They have a right to be made aware of this fact.

The classification of people who are color deficient is a complex process, and color deficient people do not all fall neatly into these categories.

There are many other color vision tests used. Sometimes lantern tests are used by the armed services, and they may be used by some other organizations which require tests. There is a Davidson and Hemmendinger Color Rule, which uses colored slides and can be used by children as young as eight years of age. (Richards, Part II) Still in use, but less frequently, is the Holmgren Yarn Test, which uses the matching of colored yarns.

In the United States, the most commonly used tests are the Ishihara, the Dvorine, and the Farnsworth tests.

The Ishihara and Dvorine tests use pseudoisochromatic (false-same color) plates. These plates have colored and gray spots in patterns which can be seen by average people but cannot be seen by the color deficient. (Richards, Part II) Red-green defects can be found using these tests but not yellow-blue.

The Farnsworth Dichotomous D-15 test was developed for industry. One of the special values of this test is that it will identify yellow-blue deficiencies as well as red-green. Colored papers are mounted in caps with numbers on the bottoms of the caps. The subject arranges the caps from the reference cap on with the next nearest color. When the caps are turned over, the numbers identify the color vision problem, if any. I know of at least one ophthalmologist who uses this test as his first choice for color vision testing. This test can be used with children from age eight on up and has been used with children as young as three.

Some researchers feel that the Farnsworth D-15 test is not adequate alone because some color deficient children can pass it. Conversely, the Ishihara and Dvorine tests do not identify some children which the Farnsworth D-15 test will identify. When testing children, a good combination is to use both a pseudoisochromatic test and the Farnsworth D-15 test.

For business and industry, the Farnsworth D-15 test is probably the most useful of the color vision tests. Too often, with a person whose color vision deficiency is so mild it causes no significant practical problem, the person is told he is color deficient because he failed a pseudoisochromatic test and he is denied employment because of the test results. Since gainful employment is crucial to most people, it would seem practical to use the Farnsworth D-15 test for all employment except for those occupations requiring a high degree of color identification . (Adams; Dreyer)

The Farnsworth Munsell 100 Hue test is a greatly expanded version of the Farnsworth D-15 test. It is used primarily for testing very fine color discrimination and is not intended as a primary color vision screening test. (Richards, Part 1,)

For testing pre-school or primary children, the Illiterate plates 18, 19, and 20 of the Ishihara series are often used. (Cox) Children are asked to trace the pathway of the number or geometric figure on the plate with their fingers or with a small, soft brush.

Testing pre-school children is not believed to produce completely satisfactory results, probably because many of the children are too immature to be able to cope adequately with test factors.

One doctor wrote that he used a mounted wall chart with pseudoisochromatic plates and suggested that patients test themselves for color deficiency. Dr. Richards (Part II) feels that in a display of that type the lighting would almost certainly be inadequate for the plates, with mixed lighting, (daylight, fluorescent light of varying kinds and sometimes with tungsten lamps) and that the doctor involved showed a lack of understanding of all the test factors.

It is important for people to know that correct lighting is absolutely essential for color vision testing. The lights recommended by the manufacturers of the tests are best. Otherwise, only north, (in the northern hemisphere) middle of the day, daylight will give proper color appearance to the testing materials. Other means of lighting the test area can distort the colors. (Richards, Part II; Farnsworth)

Testing materials not properly cared for can fade, causing alterations in colors. It is most important that the materials not be left open out in the light, but after use they should be closed and returned to the containers in which they came. Soil on the testing surfaces can also damage the colors.

In his dissertation submitted for a doctoral degree, The Development of a Low Cost Microcomputer Generated Color Vision Exam, Larry L. Bradshaw used a Commodore 64 Computer, with a General Electric 10" television set as a monitor with which he developed a color vision test. The Ishihara pseudoisochromatic plates were used to validate the study.

Bradshaw's test was designed to identify those not perceiving blue and violet as the average person does, as well as identifying those who have problems with red and green.

It was inevitable that computers would be used in this regard. I am sure that many more tests of this kind will be developed as time goes by.

The Bernell Corporation is now selling a test called The New Spectrum Color Test, which they say is specifically designed for pediatric use (ages three and up). I have seen no evaluations of this test, but it is to be hoped that it will prove to be a good one.

R. Fletcher, Professor at the City University, London, England, writes of The Fletcher-Hamblin Simplified Colour Vision Test. It consists of colored plastic squares held in plates. It can be perceived by the child as a game. The child is asked to touch the squares with colors which are 'different' from the predominant color. There is a plate which can identify yellow-blue deficiency, also. It sounds quite interesting. (For ordering, see Keeler, Ltd. in bibliography.)

Roderic W. Gillilan, O.D. of Eugene, OR, feels that a simple color vision test could be produced using colored blocks. The child could be requested to match the blocks by color (reminiscent of the Holmgren Yarn test.) I agree that this sounds like a very good idea. The test could be kept in each school and available for all kindergarten and primary school teachers to use with all their students. It is right there in early education where the color deficient child may first encounter problems.

Dr. Heath (1964) suggests a similar idea for young children. Regular wax crayons with their wrappers removed are used in the game/test. "Selecting, say, a green crayon from a box or tray of crayons of all colors, the examiner tells the child to pick out all the other crayons of the same color." This game/test should be set up so that there are at least three crayons of each color.

Of the above two test ideas, I would like to see Dr. Gillilan's developed because it would provide specific directions and information about lighting. The crayon test is a good idea, too, but I feel that many people would be careless about the type of lighting used during the test.

As stated earlier in this chapter, adequate and appropriate lighting are an important requirement for all color vision tests. If special lighting is not available, use north daylight!

The primary colors of light are red, blue and green, which create white light when added together, while red and green added together equal yellow.

Of color vision tests, the anomaloscope is the most comprehensive but is not widely used. The pseudoisochromatic (false-same color) plates are the most widely used with the Ishihara and Dvorine being most used. The Farnsworth D-15 test (using small colored caps) was developed for industry and is recommended for business and industry because it will identify all of the color deficient cases except the most mild.

In the U.S., about eight percent of human males are color deficient and about one half of one percent of human females are so affected.

Some sources (see bibliography) and prices of color vision tests:

1987

Bernell Corporation

Ishihara Color Test:	10 Plates	$60.00
	14 Plates	68.00
	24 Plates	95.00
	38 Plates	115.00

Farnsworth D-15 Color Test	$240.00
New Spectrum Color Test	$135.00
Ickikawa Igaku-Shoin	
Pseudoisochromatic Color Vision Test	$55.00

Psychological Corporation

Dvorine Color Vision Test	$159.00
Farnsworth D-15 Test for Color Blindness	$350.00

What Do the Color Deficient See?

People are usually curious about how the world looks to a color deficient person. Naturally, parents want to know what their child can see and how he sees it.

Relatives and friends of mine who are color deficient would rather not tell others they are color deficient because people often say, "What color is this? What color is that?" That can be very embarrassing as no one likes to be considered a curiosity. Lemonick says he was a reluctant hit at parties because people liked to do the same thing to him.

We can know how the world looks to the monochromat because we can see black and white movies, that's how his world appears to him. But we can never know exactly what it is like for color defecient people because we don't have their visual frame of reference and they don't have ours. In her in-depth article on what the color deficient see, Jo Ann S. Kinney says words referring to colors do not necessarily mean the same to the color deficient person as they mean to the average person. If you swim, look around underwater and notice how your own color vision has altered. (Zeltzer, 1979) You could see this better if you were swimming in a large natural water area such as a lake, river or ocean.

Looking through sun glasses of various colors is another way of seeing the world in other colors. No experiment you may try will tell you how the world looks to the color deficient, but at least, you can see the world in other colors.

The other day, I was in a sporting goods store and noticed that they had, on their sun glasses rack, some glasses with bright red lenses! I tried a pair on to see what would happen to the colors I saw, and all the trees had brown leaves! Different kinds of light alter the colors we all see, but we seldom have need to think about it. Some researechers state that reds, greens and browns are confused by many of the color deficient. (Wilson & Robinson; Dvorine) This is true for my own relatives.

In his book, *Eye and Brain*, Gregory says that he believes the color brown to be a kind of super-saturated yellow. For those people who see reds and greens as browns, it may be that brown is a version of yellow and they can distinguish yellows and blues.

Another researcher says that color deficient people mix up reds, browns, olives and golds. Many confuse purple with blue because the blue in purple is discerned but not the red. (Adams) One of my relatives told me that purple looks blue to him. Schmidt (1976) tells of a milliner who had trouble distinguishing pale blue, pink, violet and lavender from blue-green.

(See chapter on, Tests For Color Vision, for explanation of different varieties of color vision deficiency.)

The anamalous trichromat is able to see more color than the dichromat, though both types of deficiency produce many of the same problems in varying degrees. For those dichromats with protanopia (about one per cent of the color deficient), red appears black. (Setright) Unfortunately, many public signs have red letters on a black or very dark background. It is equally unfortunate when the color deficient have to try to see red on green or green on red, or either one on brown, unless there is considerable contrast between the message and the background.

Most of our traffic lights are somewhat different now than they were many decades ago. Blue has been added to the green and yellow has been added to the red. (Goldstein & Borreson) Now most color deficient people can distinguish these lights. Also, the red light is usually on top and the green on the bottom unless they are side by side. Then the red is to the left and the green to the right. (Traffic Engineering Div., Eugene, Oregon) Many states now require yellow for school buses, because yellow is easily visible to nearly everyone. (Rosenberg)

Color deficient people are often able to detect camouflage which is invisible to the average person because artificial camouflage is created to confuse the average observer. (Kalmus) During World War II, color deficient persons were used in the military to spot camouflage. (Wright) They now have electronic and photographic means of camouflage detection. I have found that some color deficient people can also detect natural camouflage used by animals. That very observant mother, Shirley Rosenberg, in her article, "The Boy Who Thought Pancakes Were Green," writes that her son could spot lizards, toads and injured birds more easily than other people. I know a man who worked with a color deficient forester, and that forester is also good at spotting natural camouflage.

A woman acquaintance and my own brother have told me that the green 'go' lights look white to them.

The color deficient person cannot really tell you how he sees colors because he is looking at a world colored differently than your world. Parents can learn some things by unobtrusive observation. A group of color deficient people may each see the world somewhat differently from each other.

For the color deficient, words referring to color do not have the same meaning as those words have for the average person.

I believe it really requires trying to use one's imagination to even begin to understand how the world may appear to color deficient people. Also, I don't believe we should ever become smug enough to think we 'know' just what they see.

How We See

As I'm sure you know, in pitch darkness we can see nothing at all. Our eyes must have light in order to see. In order to distinguish colors, adequate light is essential. For instance, if you were to go outside at night where there was no auxilary lighting, you would see the world in shades of gray. It is a fact that different kinds of light will alter the perception of any given color. Try looking at the same colors under sunlight, flourescent light, incandescent light, and different types of street lights. See how the colors appear to change.

Light is part of the electromagnetic spectrum, but only a very small part. You can see by the diagram of that spectrum, that there are various kinds of energy which affect our daily lives in many ways even though most of that spectrum is invisible to us. (Reinfeld ; Cruz-Coke)

The region of the electromagnetic spectrum which is visible to the human eye runs from the region of the color red through orange, yellow, green, blue, and violet light regions. But, actually, the human eye does not see all the colors in the color spectrum. We do not see pure red nor pure purple. They fall into the infra-red and the ultra-violet ranges and our retinas are not able to utilize these colors. (Cruz-Coke)

Long electric waves
Long radio waves
Standard broadcast
Radio short waves
Television and radar bands
Infrared or heat rays
Visible range
Ultraviolet rays
X-rays
Gamma rays

The electromagnetic spectrum, ranging from waves of the lowest energy, lowest frequency and greatest length (at the top) up to the waves of greatest energy, highest frequency and shortest length (at the bottom). (Reinfeld)

While humankind is making ever increasing use of the electromagnetic spectrum, our lives revolve around the visible portion of that spectrum.

We obtain a great deal of our knowledge about the world through our eyes and the human eye could well be considered our most useful and complex organ. Still, to this day, we do not completely understand all the functions of the eye.

On the outside, the human eye is covered by the sclera. (a.) The so-called 'white' of the eye is part of this sclerotic covering. The transparent cornea (b.) through which we see is also part of the sclera. The cornea covers the iris (c.) and pupil (d.) and admits light to the interior of the eye. Behind the cornea is a space filled with a clear, limpid

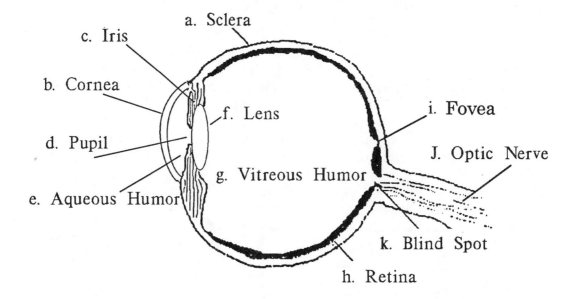

fluid called the aqueous humor (e.). The iris is the opaque, muscular curtain which is suspended in the aqueous humor in front of the lens. The iris is deeply pigmented (from very pale blue to very dark brown) to exclude the entrance of light and there is a hole in the center which is called the pupil. The pupil looks black but that is only because no light is reflected back out of the eye. Next comes the crystaline lens, (f.) which is both transparent and elastic.

The lens changes shape to accomodate both near and far vision. The large rear portion of the eyeball is filled with a colorless, transparent jelly called the vitreous humor (g.) The inner back part of the eyeball is lined by the retina. (h.) (Freese; Hammond; Colliers Encyclopedia) R. L. Gregory states that the retina is a special part of the brain which has budded out and become sensitive to light.

There are two kinds of light-receiving cells in the retina, called rods and cones. The rod cells are long and thin and the cone cells are shorter and thicker. The cone cells are, in fact, shaped like tiny cones. (Begbie; Gregory;Freese) There is a pigment in the rods called rhodopsin. One theory about rhodopsin says that it is sensitive to all light but shows all light in shades of gray. The rods function under low illumination and give us our night vision. Only rods are in the outer areas of the retina, so the rods also give us our side or peripheral vision. The human retina has more than one hundred million rods and cones, but there are nearly eighteen times as many rods as cones. (National Soc. for the Prevention of Blindness; Begbie)

Cones give us our color vision. These cones are located toward the center of the retina. In fact, they increase in number until at the retinal center there is a small area called the fovea (i) which is composed entirely of cones. This is the area which gives us our sharpest vision. (Gregory) The place where the optic nerve enters is called the 'blind spot', (k.) a tiny spot on the retina not affected by light. (Webster's Third New International Dictionary)

There is a light-sensitive substance in the cones called iodopsin and it is theorized that it is iodopsin that enables the cones to respond to color. The rhodopsin in the rods and iodopsin in the cones produce nerve signals when light hits them. These signals go to connector cells and on up the optic nerve (j) to the brain. (Collier's Encyclopedia)

There are many different theories which try to explain the phenomena of how we see color. None of the theories so far are a final answer because none accounts for all aspects of color vision. (Judd, 1975)

Through human history there have always been a few people who were aware of color vision deficiency. The first recorded suggestion that colors do not necessarily appear the same to everyone comes from the time of Plato. A few studies were also done on the subject as early as the sixteen and seventeen hundreds.

In 1794, John Dalton was the first person to really study the phenomena of color vision deficiency. (Patterson) Dalton, a famous English chemist, physicist and mathematics teacher has been called 'the father of the atomic theory'. (Patterson) Both he and his brother were color deficient. He believed that color deficiency was caused by a problem with the fluids in the eyeball. For a century afterwards, the problem was usually referred to as 'daltonism' and is still referred to by that term in French and Spanish speaking countries. (Kalmus)

Thomas Young first suggested a theory of color vision in 1807. He supposed that there are three mechanisms in the retina associated with red, green and violet. It is called the trichromatic theory.

Herman von Helmholtz, in mid-nineteenth century, altered Young's theory in order to account for color vision deficiency. He theorized that color deficiency is due to a lack of one of the three primary color sensitive functions of the cones. For protanopia, the 'red' is missing, for deuteranopia, the 'green', and for tritanopia, the 'violet'. (Mueller, Rudolph) These theories have been combined and are called the Young-Helmholtz theory.

In 1872, Karl Hering stressed the psychology of color perception. He theorized that the retina's receptors are mere absorbers of light and that color discrimination begins in the coding mechanisms located farther along the optic system. Hering theorized that while most of the coding mechanisms send only black and white signals to the brain, two other types react to color in an odd way. One sends signals for either red or green and the other for either blue or yellow. He believed that these color coders had to 'shut off' green to send a red signal and vice versa and the same with blue and yellow. This is referred to as an opponent process theory. Hering felt that color deficiency was due to a nerve structure defect beyond the retina along the visual pathway. Some researchers now feel that there are probably factors in both the Young-Helmholtz theory and the Hering theory that are correct. (Mueller, Rudolph)

Edwin Land, who invented the Land camera, made a fascinating discovery while experimenting with photography. He found that if he took two black and white pictures of the same scene, one through a red filter and one through a green filter, super imposed the two negatives and shone a yellow light through them, the result was a picture that, while pale, was in all its natural colors!

From this beginning, Land developed his Retinex Theory of color vision involving the retina-and-cortex system (retinex). Land theorizes that light rays are bearers of information that the eye uses to give colors to objects. The eye perceives colors by comparing longer and shorter wavelengths of light. (Land, 1977)

Since this material is not intended to cover extensively all the information on the theories of the causes of color vision deficiency, I will just say that other theories exist and more of them will be developed. In time, there will probably be absolute proof of why some of us are color deficient, but to my knowledge, that proof does not yet exist.

We must have light in order to see and our perception of the world revolves around the light and the lights that, at least somewhat, govern our activities. The pathway from the eye to the brain and the brain itself are involved with our color vision. How our eyes see color, and why some of us do not see all the colors, are subjects of great interest and, as yet, they produce more questions than answers.

Treatment

Over the years, many different methods of treating color deficient people have been tried.

Some people have claimed that vitamin A has cured their color deficiency. The vitamin may improve visual acuity but, it has no proven effect on color deficiency. (Ruch)

Scores of methods for training persons with deficient color vision have been developed, often with claims of considerable improvement. Usually, training consists of a great deal of practice in naming colored items or lights. Sometimes, the subjects' eyes have been exposed to strong, colored lights. (Heath, 1974) But no amount of 'training' enables a color deficient person to pass color vision tests any better than they could before 'training'.

I once knew an excellent teacher who was convinced that she had been able to 'train' students out of color deficiency. Of course, her 'trained' students were not tested by a vision specialist after her efforts, but she, herself, was convinced that they were no longer color deficient. In her defense, she was at least aware of them and tried to do something about their problem and that is more help than most color deficient children receive.

Not a single authentic case of actual change in the color vision of any color deficient person has been documented. Kessler; Judd & Wyszechi (1963), and Mantz all agree on this. Any apparent improvement is simply that the color deficient person has learned to pick up other clues from the objects used in the training. In some cases, apparent improvement was a result of the learning of color names by normal persons who were uneducated as to color names.

The physical vision system of the color deficient person is simply not able to incorporate the colors in which he is deficient any more than the rest of us can see into the ultra violet range where the humming bird and the bee can see a color invisible to us.

The use of colored filters for aiding color deficient people was proposed as far back as 1837. (Paulson) There were early attempts at improving color vision by using filters, lights, prisms, and other things.

A red filter will darken greens and will give reds a vibrancy or luster as though polished. Any colored filter over one eye will produce a peculiar luster or sheen on some colored objects. (Siegel) A red filter or lens will not enable the color deficient person to see reds and greens as the average person does but will usually enable him to tell them apart. (Paulson; Kernell)

The X-Chrom lens is a recent addition to these endeavors. It is a corneal contact lens transmitting light in the red zone. It is worn on only one eye. This lens is an all red, hard contact lens and is usually obvious to the observer, unless the wearer has very dark eyes. Some people may be embarrassed at appearing in public with one red eye. Dr. Zeltzer, who patented the X-Chrom lens, has many case records of people who say they have been helped by the red lens. Some people are able to pass the Ishihara color vision test when wearing the lens when they could not do so without it. This has apparently been of benefit to a considerable number of people in their working life as well as in their private life. (X-Chrom Lens: Case Reports)

When a person puts any colored lens on or before one eye, one of the effects is called the Pulfrich Effect, or the Pulfrich Phenomenon. It results in the apparent distortion of some observed motion. Zeltzer says that people do adapt to this effect. Another researcher states that of the subjects he tested, some did adapt and some did not. (Siegel)

At Univ. College in Wales, in studies done on binocular filters as an aid for the color deficient, Wilson and Robinson tested a somewhat different method. They found that J.C. Maxwell, in 1885, had suggested using a red filter over one eye and a green over the other, though he did not carry the experiment through. Others have experimented with this idea. (Schmidt, 1976) Wilson and Robinson state that both Maxwell's red filter and the X-Chrom lens cut down on all light entering the eye except red and a green filter cuts down on all light except green. This cuts down on the visibility of other colors seen by the eye and this is not recommended. In order to avoid this they used filters which stopped red and stopped green. A cyan (greenish) filter was used to stop red and a magenta (reddish) filter to stop green. Filters of these kinds are used for color photography. These do not cut down on the other light (colors) entering the eye except for yellow. Apparently, a colored lens over each eye eliminates the Pulfrich Effect as none was mentioned. The glasses they used proved to provide a definite, though limited, aid to color vision. I have corresponded with these researchers. They report recently that they have not done any further work as they had not been able to find a suitable dye for the lenses. They were using glasses, not contact lenses.

More recently, in the U.S., Jay L. Schlanger has developed the JLS lens, both in a magenta (reddish) and in an aqua (greenish) tinted, soft contact lens. As with the X-Chrom lens, many of the subjects wearing the JLS lens were able to pass the pseudoisochromatic color vision tests. With both the X-Chrom lens and the JLS lenses, subjects report enhanced enjoyment of colors, and improvement in matching colors (as with their clothes).

I have corresponded with Dr. Schlanger and find that he uses both a greenish and a reddish lens in his work with color deficient patients. He reports that most people feel that they get the best color vision effect with a red lens alone. Also, he does put the colored part of the lens right over the pupil and therefore the lens is not as obvious to the observer.

He does not feel that school children should wear colored lenses. Instead, their teachers and parents should be aware of their color vision problems.

Dr. Schlanger is producing only soft contact lenses. These can be made in prescription lenses. However, these lenses cannot be made for corrections of all vision problems, astigmatism, for instance. However, a patient could use the lens and also wear a pair of prescription glasses.

If a patient wishes a JLS lens, Dr. Schlanger recommends that the doctor obtain a colored filter, Kodak Wratten #30, catalog number 1495639. Have the patient hold this filter in front of one eye and see if it helps his color vision. If so, contact Dr. Schlanger. The lens can be obtained through him.
Jay L. Schlanger, O.D., Cedars-Sinai Medical Tower, 8631 W.
Third St., Suite 800-E, Los Angeles, CA 90048

Dr. John E. Perkins of Eugene, OR (who has prescribed contact lenses for children) sees no problem with children wearing a colored contact lens for aiding a color vision problem, providing the parents understand the situation and the child is reasonably accepting. (Dr. Perkins and Dr. Gillilan are in the Family Vision Center in Eugene, OR.)

Dr. Harry Zeltzer, who produced the X-Chrom lens, has now produced a new X-Chrom soft contact lens. It is not on the market yet (Sept.,1988), but should be soon.

Richer and Adams are doing in depth research on colored lenses. One of their articles discusses extensive testing using the X-Chrom lens, X-Chrom paddle (in color, similar to the X-Chrom lens), and Kodak Wratten no. 30 filter. These are red and pink filters. They believe their work will aid in the design of new filters which might be developed for specific categories of the color deficient.

Valley Contax of Eugene, OR produces a red contact lens (Rhoda-LUX lens) which is less expensive than many of the other colored lenses.

Work with colored contact lenses would appear to offer for the first time some real help to those with color deficient vision. While there is no cure these approaches at least offer some significant help.

SOURCES:

Family Vision Center, 1471 Pearl St., Eugene, OR 97401

Valley Contax, 1310 Coburg Road, Eugene, OR 97401

Dr. Harry Zeltzer, X-Chrom Division, Young Contact Lens Laboratories, 1050 Commonwealth

Bibliography for Color Vision Deficiency

Adams, Anthony J., O. D., Ph. D. Color Vision Testing in Optometric Practice. *Journal of the American Optometric Association* v. 45, no. 1 Jan., 1974 pp.35-42

American Optometric Association pamphlet *Do You Know These Facts About Colorblindness?*

Basford, Adelphia Meyer. *Is the Child Color-Blind?* The Delta Kappa Gamma Bulletin Spring, 1976 pp. 49-52

Begbie, G. Hugh. *Seeing and the Eye; An Introduction to Vision.* Published for; The American Museum of Natural History, Natural History Press, Garden City, New York c1969

Bradshaw, Larry L. *Development of a Low Cost Microcomputer Generated Color Vision Exam* Dissertation, Iowa State Univ., Ames, Iowa 1984

Burnham, Robert W., Comptrollers Div., Eastman Kodak Co.; Hanes, Randall M., Applied Physics Laboratory, Johns Hopkins University Bartleson, C. James, Research Laboratories, Eastman Kodak Co. *Color: A Guide to Basic Facts and Concepts A report of the Inter-Society Color Sub-Committee for Problem 20 Basic Elements of Color Education* John Wiley and Sons, Inc. c1963

Cobb, Stephen R. *Evidence for an Effect by Colour Defect on Personality Perceptual and Motor Skills* v. 51, Aug.,1981 pp.159-66

Cox, Brian J., M. Ed., D.O.S. Validity of a Preschool Colour Vision Test *Journal of School Health* March, 1971 pp. 163-165

Cruz-Coke, Ricardo, M. D. *Color Blindness, An Evolutionary Approach Charles* C. Thomas, Pub. Springfield, Ill., U.S.A. c1970

Davids, Richard C. Confessions of a Color-Blind Male. *Reader's Digest* Aug., 1962 pp. 187-92

Dreyer, V. Occupational Possibilities of Colour Defectives *ACTA Ophthalmologica* 1969 v.47 p.523

Dvorine, Israel, M.D. Can Your Child See Red? *Child Study* Spring, 1958 XXXV No. 2 pp. 40-1

Dvorine, Israel M.D. *Color Vision Test*

Espinda, Stanley D., Ph.D. Color Vision Deficiency: A Learning Disability? *Journal of Learning Disabilities* v.6 No.3 March, 1973 pp.42-4, 166

The Eye. *Collier's Encyclopedia* Macmillan Educational Corp.,N.Y. v.9 1980 p.514

Farnsworth, Dean. *Farnsworth Dichotomous Test for Color Blindness Manual by Dean Farnsworth for Panel D-15* c1947

Fletcher, R. The Fletcher-Hamblin Simplified Colour Vision Test *The Optician* 1984 v. 187, pp.29-31

Freese, Arthur S. *The Miracle of Vision* Harper and Row, Pub. N.Y. c.1977

Gillilan, Roderick W., O.D. 1471 Pearl St. Eugene, OR 97401

Goldsmith, Timothy H. Yale Univ. Hummingbirds See Near Ultraviolet Light *Science* v.207 Feb. 15, 1980 pp.786-8

Goldstein, A.G., Borresen, C.R.Red-Green Color Deficiency and Compensatory Learning: an Experimental Critique *American Journal of Psychology* Sept., 1960 pp. 482-5

Gregory, Richard Langton. *Eye and Brain; The Psychology of Seeing.* World Univ. Library McGraw-Hill Book Co. c1966

Guidelines for Developing Eye Health Programs for Children. National Association of Vision Program Consultants. 1775 Church St., N.W. Washington, D.C. 20036. Jan., 1981

Hammond, Winifred. *The Story of Your Eye.* Coward, McCann and Geoghegan, Inc., N.Y. c1975

Heath, Gordon G. Color Vision. *Vision of Children, an Optometric Symposium* Hirsch, Monroe J.,O.D.,Ph.D., Wick, Ralph E.,O.D., editors Chilton Books N.Y. and Phildelphia c1964 pp.291-309

Heath, Gordon G., O.D., Ph.D. The Handicap of Color Blindness. *Journal of the American Optometric Association* v.45 No.1 Jan., 1974 pp.62-69

Johnson, Martin. Color Defectiveness: A Personal Account *Orthomolecular Psychiatry* 1980 v.9, No.1 pp.21-23

Jonas, Doris; Jonas, David. *Other Senses, Other Worlds.* Stein, and Day, Pub., N.Y. c1975

Judd, Deane B.; Wyszecki, Gunter. *Color in Business, Science and Industry 2nd ed.* John Wiley & Sons, N.Y. c1963

Judd, Deane B.; Wyszecki, Gunter. *Color in Business, Science and Industry 3rd ed.* John Wiley & Sons, N.Y. c1975

Kalmus, H., Sc.D., M.D. *Diagnosis and Genetics of Defective Colour Vision.* Pergamon Press London and N.Y., etc. c1965

Kernell, D. Dept. of Neurophysiology, Univ. of Amsterdam Eerste Coinbst. Huygensstraat 20, Amsterdam, The Netherlands. A Simple and Inexpensive Method for Helping 'Red-Green' Blind Subjects to Identify Colours Physiological Society, *Journal of Physiology (London)* June, 1974 p.73P

Kessler, Julius, M.D. What Can Be Done For the Color Blind? *Annals of Ophthalmology* April, 1977 9 (4):431-3

Kinney, Jo Ann S. Color Defectives - Basic Facts on What These Individuals See *Color Engineering* March/April 1971 pp.19-24

Lampe, John M., M.D.; Doster, Mildred E., M.D.; Beal, Barry B. Summary of a Three-Year Study of Academic and School Achievement Between Color-Deficient and Normal Primary Age Pupils: Phase Two *Journal of School Health* May, 1973 v.XLIII No.5

Land, Edwin H. Retinex Theory of Color Vision *Scientific American* Dec., 1977 p.108

Lemonick, Michael. Are You Color Blind? *Science Digest* Jan., 1984 pp.74-7

Lewis, Jan. Keeping an Eye on Color Blindness. *Current Health* April, 1986 pp.22-3

Litton, Freddie W. Color Vision Deficiency in LD Children. *Academic Therapy* March, 1979 pp.437-43

Lyle, William M., O.D., Ph.D. Drugs and Conditions Which May Affect Color Vision, Part I *Journal of the American Optometric Association* v.45 No.1 Jan., 1974 pp.47-60

Lyle, W. M., O.D., Ph.D.Drugs and Conditions Which May Affect Color Vision, Part II *Journal of the American Optometric Association* v.45 No.2 Feb., 1974 p.173-82

Mantz, Genelle Keithly, B.S. Supervisor of Nurses, Dist. 64, Park Ridge-Niles, Illinois Conditioning or Retraining Color-Blind. *Journal of School Health* April, 1969 39:275-6

March of Dimes Birth Defects Foundation. 1275 Mamaroneck Ave. White Plains, N.Y. 10605

Mueller, Conrad G.; Rudolph, Mae, and the editors of Life. *Light and Vision.* Time, Inc., N.Y. c1966 pp.119-25

Nagy, Allen L.; MacLeod, Doanld I.A.; Heyneman, Nicholas E.; Eisner, Alvin Four Cone Pigments in Women Heterozygous for Color Deficiency. *Optical Society of America* June, 1981 v.71 No.6 pp. 719-22

National Society For the Prevention of Blindness. *Color Vision Sight Saving Review* Winter, 1959 pp.197-203

O'Neill, Mary. *Hailstones and Halibut Bones* Doubleday Garden City, N.Y. c1961

Patterson, Elizabeth C. *John Dalton and the Atomic Theory.* Doubleday & Co.,Inc. Garden City, N.Y. c1970 pp.60-65

Paulson, Helen M. Description of the X-Chrom Lens (Evaluation). *Military Medicine* Aug.,1980 145 (8):557-60

Peters, George A. Color Blindness. *Exceptional Children* XXXII No.6 March, 1957 pp.241-5

Pickford, R. W. A Deuteranomalous Artist. British *Journal of Psychology* 1964 v.55 (4) pp.469-76

Pickford, R.W. *Individual Differences in Colour Vision.* Routledge and Kegan Paul Ltd. London c1951

Reinfeld, Fred. Rays, *Visible and Invisible.* Sterling Pub. Co., N.Y. c1958

Renaldo, John M., O.D. Usefulness of Color Vision Testing and Color Fields. *Journal of the American Optometric Association* Nov.,1977 v.48 No.11 p.1411

Richards, Oscar, Ph.D. Practical Color Vision Testing in the Optometric Office Part I *Oregon Optometrist* Summer, 1978 pp.7-9

Richards, Oscar, Ph.D. Practical Color Vision Testing in the Optometric Office Part II *Oregon Optometrist* Fall, 1978

Richer, Stuart; Adams, Anthony J. April,1984 An Experimental Test of Filter-Aided Dichromatic Color Discrimination *American Journal of Optometry and Physiological Optics* v.61(4) 256-64

Rosenberg, Shirley Sirota. The Boy Who Thought Pancakes Were Green *Parents Magazine* Feb., 1963 pp.70-l, 145-6

Ruch, F. L. *Psychology and Life*. Scott, Foresman, Chicago c1963

Sassenrath, Julius M.; Pierce, Lajla C.; Maddux, Robert E.Functional Color Components Used in Reading Instruction. *Psychology in the Schools* Jan., 1979 pp.132-6

Schlanger, Jay L. The JLS Lens: An Aid for Patients with Color Vision Problems. *American Journal of Optometry and Physiological Optics* Feb., 1985 v.62 (2) pp.149-51

Schmidt, Ingeborg, M.D. Prof.emer.,Sch. of Opoto.,Indiana Univ. June/July, 1976 Visual Aids For Correction of Red-Green Colour Deficiencies *Canadian Journal of Optometry*, v.38,#2, pp.38-47

Setright, L.J.K. The Eye of the Beholder. *Car and Driver* Aug.,1978

Sewell, Julia H. Color Counts, Too. *Academic Therapy* Jan.,1983 18:3 pp.329-36

Sharp, Evelyn. *Parent's Guide to the New Mathematics*. E.P. Dutton & Co., Inc. N.Y. c1964

Shearron, Gilbert F., Jr., Ed.D. George Peabody College for Teachers, Nashville, Tenn. *The Intelligence, Socio-economic Status, and Reading Achievement of Color Deficient Primary School Children*. Dissertation, May, 1964

Shearron, Gilbert F., Ed.D. Color Vision Deficiency in Primary School Children *Sight Saving Review* Fall, 1965 v.34-36 No.3 pp.148-150

Shute, Donald T.,O.D.; Oshinskie, Leonard, O.D. Acquired Color Vision Defects and Self Monitoring of Blood Sugar in Diabetics. *Journal of the American Optometric Association* v.57 No.11 Nov.,1986 pp.825-31

Siegel, Irwin M., Ph.D. X-Chrom Lens: On Seeing Red. *Survey of Ophthalmology* v.25 No.5 March-April, 1981 pp.312-23

Snyder, C.R., Ph.D. Psychological Implications of Being Color Blind. *Journal of Special Education* Spring, 1973 v.7 No.1 pp.51-4

Stone, Irving. *Love Is Eternal*. Doubleday & Co.,Inc. Garden City, N.Y. c1954 p.377

Thuline, Horace C., M.D. Color-Vision Defects in American School Children. *Journal of the American Medical Association* May 11, 1964 188:514-8

Vision Screening Guidlines for School Nurses National Association for School Nurses , Inc. Box 1300, Scarborough, ME 04074

Volpe, E. Peter. *Understanding Evolution*. Wm.C. Brown Co., Pub. Dubuque, Iowa c1967 p.29

Waddington, Mary, Lecturer in Child Development Univ. of London Inst. of Education Colour Blindness in Young Children. *Educational Research* June, 1965 7:236-40

Walls, Gordon L.; Mathews, Ravenna W. *New Means of Studying Color Blindness and Normal Foveal Color Vision* Univ. of California Press Berleley & L.A. 1952 p.25

Wildman, Peggy Riggs Dept. of Education of the Graduate School, George Peabody College for Teachers, Nashville, Tenn. *Teacher Awareness of Color Deficiency and Its Effect on Instruction in the First Grade.* Dissertation Aug., 1964

Willis, Judith. Genetic Counseling: Learning What to Expect. *FDA Consumer,* Official magazine of the FDA Rockville, MA

Wilson, J. A.; Robinson, J. O. Binocular Filters as an Aid to Color Discrimination by Dichromats. *American Journal of Optometry and Physiol. Optics* Dec.,1980 v.57 No.12 pp.893-901

Wright, W. D. *Researches on Normal and Defective Colour Vision.* Henry Kempton London c1946

The X-Chrom Lens: Case Reports. *Journal of the American Optometric Assoc.* Jan., 1974 pp.81-7

The X-Chrom Manual. X-Chrom Corp. staff under supervision of
Dr. Harry I. Zeltzer c1975

Zaba, Joel N., M.A.,O.D.Color Deficiency, Optometry and Education. *Journal of the American Optometric Assoc.* Jan.,1974 v.,45 no.1 p.94

Supplemental Reading
Materials on Color Vision

A Partial List of Articles on Color Coded Learning Materials:

Althouse, Rosemary; Main, Cecil. Science Learning Center: Hub of Science Activities *Childhood Education* v. 50 Fall, 1974 p.222

Bidwell, James K., Math Dept., Central Michigan University, Mt. Pleasant, Mich. Number Sentence Trios *Arithmetic Teacher* v. 21 Feb.,1974 pp. 150-2

Bruno, Golden B., Ed. D.; Cutler, Barbara Learning With Wooden Blocks *Exceptional Parent* v. 9:A Feb.,1979 pp. 30-1

Colburn, Candace. Through Color Coding *Instructor* Nov.,1971 p.60

Cox, Anne Mae. Magic While They Are Young *The Arithmetic Teacher* March, 1974 pp. 178-81

Ewbank, William A. The Use of Color for Teaching Mathematics. *Arithmetic Teacher* Sept., 1978 pp.53-7

Green, Roberta, Dover Public Schools, Dover, Mass.A Color-coded Method of Teaching Basic Arithmetic Concepts and Procedures. *Arithmetic Teacher* March, 1970 pp.231-3

Holan, Edith. Get Color in Early *Instructor* June, 1970 p.60

Otto, Wayne, Ph.D., Askov, Eunice, M.A. Role of Color in Learning and Instruction *Journal of Special Education* Winter, 1968 pp.155-65

Payne, Sara. Explaining Music to Children by Color. *Times Educational Supplement (U.K.)* June 5, 1970 p.86

Perrin, Mary Jane. Grade Level Color Coding. *Journal of Reading* Nov., 1972 p.159

Prater, Mildred Juanita. *Color Uses in Primary Instructional Materials and Possible Implications for Color Deficient Children.* Dissertation, George Peabody College for Teachers, Nashville, Tennessee (Vanderbilt U.) Aug., 1967

Vail, Patricia, Reading Specialist 15 Reading Games You Can Adapt to Any Level *Instructor* Oct.,1976 v.86 pt.1 pp.60-2

Wohl, Jane E. Color Sets: Learning Colors is in the Cards. *Learning* Oct., 1980 p.60

46

Additional materials of possible interest:

(AIC) Bulletin Apprenticeship Information Center State of Oregon Employment Division Department of Human Resources Bulletin # 23

Barker, Donald G. Color Perception Requirements of 4,000 Jobs *Journal of Employment Counseling* March, 1971

Beacham, Ruby C.,R.N.; Hisle, Margaret C., R.N., M. Ed. A Color-Blind Testing Program in the Baltimore City Public Schools *Journal of School Health* Dec., 1965 35:460-6

Birren, Faber. *Color and Human Response* Litton Educational Publishing, Inc. Van Nostrand Reinhold Co., N. Y. c. 1978

Bixby, William *Waves, Pathways of Energy.* David McKay and Co., Inc. N.Y. c. 1963

Bourges, Jean, President of the Bourges Color Corp., New York, N. Y. You Can Only See Color Straight Ahead *American Artist* Oct., 1982 p. 10

Breton, Michael E., Ph. D.; Nelson, Leonard B., M.D. What Do Color Blind Children Really See? Guidelines for Clinical Prescreening Based on Recent Findings *Survey of Ophthalmology* v.27, no. 5 March-April, 1983 pp. 306-12

Buck, George E. *Colour-Blindness in the Laboratory (Letter).* Clinical Laboratory, University of Texas Medical Branch. Galveston, Texas, U.S.A. The Lancet, April 12, 1980

Cavalli-Sforza, L.L., Bodner, W. F. *Genetics of Human Populations (A chapter on X-Linked Polymorphisms)* W. H. Freeman and Co., San Francisco, Cal. c1971

Cobb, Stephen R. *A Study of the Normal Colour Vision of Art Students* Dept. of Psychology, Univ. of Glasgow 1971

Color Vision Deficiencies in Youths 12-17 Years of Age *United States DHEW Pub. No. (HRA) 74-1616* January, 1974

Dannenmaier, W. D., Drury College The Effect of Color Perception on Success in High School Biology *Journal of Experimental Education* Winter, 1972 v. 41, no. 2 pp.15-17

Dogigli, Johannes. *The Magic of Rays* Translated from the German and edited by Charles Fullman Alfred A. Knopf N. Y. c1957

Dorst, Jean *The Life of Birds vol. 1* Translated by I. C. J. Galbraith. Columbia Univ. Press N. Y. c1971

Dwyer, Francis M. Color as an Instructional Variable. *AV Communication Review* v. 19 No. 4 Winter, 1971 pp 399-416

Dwyer, Francis M., Lamberski, Richard J. A Review of the Research on the Effects of the Use of color in the Teaching-Learning Process *International Journal of Instructional Media* v. 10(4), 1982-83 pp. 303-27

Edge, Ronald D., Ph.D. Color Blindness *Physics Teacher* April, 1983 pp.264 & 26

Edge, R.D.; Jones, Edwin R. Demonstrating Additive Primary Colors. *Physics Teacher* May, 1984 pp.320-3

Eliot, Alexander. Did Monet See What He Thought He Saw? *Atlantic.* Dec., 1973 pp.108-111

Engel, Leonard. *New Genetics* Doubleday & Co., Inc. Garden City, N.Y. c1967

Enright, J. T. Distortions of Apparent Velocity: A New Optical Illusion *Science,* 1970 168: 464-7

Espinda, Stanley D., Ph.D.*Color Vision Deficiency in Third and Sixth Grade Boys in Association to Academic Achievement and Descriptive Behavioral Patterns* Dissertation, Univ. of Southern California, 1971

Feallock, J. Bennett; Southard, Jack F.; Kobayashi, M.; Howell, William C., Ohio State University. Absolute Judgement of Colors in the Federal Standards System *Journal of Applied Psychology* v.50 No.3 1966 pp.266-72

Goodman, Mark D., Ph.D.; Cundick, Bert P., Ph.D.Learning Rates With Black and Colored Letters *Journal of Learning Disabilities* Nov., 1976 pp.68-70

Graham, Ben V., F.S.M.C., Ph.D. Mechanisms of Color Vision. *Journal of the American Optometric Association* v.45 No..1 Jan., 1974

Grether, Walter F. Color Vision and Color Blindness in Monkeys. Johns Hopkins Press, [Baltimore, Maryland] *Comparative Psychology Monographs* Serial N. 76 v.15 No.4 June,1939

Grunberg, Eleanor M., R.N., F.A.S.H.A. Color Deficient Versus Color Blind *Journal of School Health* v.XLIII No.20 p.135

Haas, George H. The Orange That Lets You Get Your Buck. *Outdoor Life* Sept., 1981 pp.64 and 74

Halberstein, Robert A., Crawford, Michael H. Anomalous Color Vision in Three Mexican Populations *American Journal of Phys. Anthropology* v.15 1974 pp.91-4

Heel, A.C.S. van; Velzel, C.H.F. *What Is Light?* World Univ. Library McGraw-Hill Book Co. N.Y. c1968

Howard, A.H. Colour Blind Drivers of Motot Vehicles (Three letters from different people) *Canadian Medical Association Journal* March 22, 1980 p.638

Ichikawa, Hiroshi; Majima, Akio. Dept. of Ophthalmology of the Central Hospital of the Japanese National Railways and the Nagoya City Univ. Medical School, Tokyo, Japan. Genealogical Studies on Interesting Families of Defective Colour Vision Discovered by a Mass Examination in Japan and Formosa. *Modern Problems Ophthal.* 1974 13 (0) :265-71

Justen, Joseph E. III, Ed.D.; Harth, Robert, Ed.D. Relationship Between Figure-Ground Discrimination and Color Blindness in Learning Disabled Children. *Journal of Learning Disabilities* Feb., 1976 pp.43-6

Kavner, Richard S., O.D.; Dusky, Lorrainbe *Total Vision.* A. and W. Pub., Inc., N.Y. c1978

Knafle, June D. Word Perception: Cues Aiding Structure Detection. (Condensation of a Ph.D. Dissertation -Eastern Connecticut State College) *Reading Research Quarterly* Summner, 1973 pp.502-23

Knight, Dunlap , Univ. of Cal., Los Angeles Defective Color Vision and Its Remedy *Journal of Comparative Psychology* April, 1945 v.37-38

Kronfeld, Peter C., M.D. *Human Eye in Anatomical Transparencies.* Bausch & Lomb Press, N.Y. c1943

Lamberski, Richard J.; Dwyer, Francis M. Instructional Effect of Coding (Color and Black and White) on Information Acquisition and Retrieval *Educational Communication and Technology* v.31 No.1 pp.9-12

Lampe, John M., M.D. An Evaluative Study of Color-Vision Tests for Kindergarten and First Grade Pupils *Journal of School Health* May, 1969

Land, Edwin H. Experiments in Color Vision *Scientific American* May, 1959 pp.84-95

Linksz, Arthur L.Improvement of Color Vision . *American Journal of Ophthalmology* June, 1966 61:1553-4

Linne, Andrea Now, in Living Color *Family Health* March, 1981 p.20

Lockmiller, Pauline; Di Nello, Mario C. Texas A.& M. Univ. Words in Color Versus a Basal Reader Program *With Retarded Readers in Grade 2 Journal of Educational Research* v.63 No.7 March, 1970 pp.330-4

Logan, J.S., M.D., F.R.C.P. The Red-Green Blind Eye. *Practitioner* v.226 May, 1982 pp.879-83 (U.K. publication)

Lorenz, Alice B.; McClure, William E. The Influence of Color Blindness on Intelligence and Achievement of College Men *Journal of Applied Psychology* 1935 v.19

MacLennan, Munr *Secret of Oliver Goldsmith* Vantage Press N.Y. c1975

Marlow, Sonja Federal Color Vision Requirements, Compilation derived from the 'Handbook of Federal Vision Requirements and Information' H.E. Mahlman, Professional Press *Submitted for publication in the Journal of the Am. Optometric Association* Oct., 1973

Millodot, Michel, Ph.D.; Lamont, Anne, B. Appl. Sc. Colour Vision Deficiencies in French Canadian School Children. *Canadian Journal of Public Health* Nov.-Dec.,1974 v.65

Moses, Robert A. *Adler's Physiology of the Eye - Clinical Applications 5th ed.* The C.V. Mosby Co. c1970 p.532, p.635

Pearl, Sydney S. Color Defective Individuals (letter). *Am. Journal of Ophthalmology* May, 1978 85(5-Pt.1) 722-3

Pease, Paul L., O.D., Ph.D. Clinical Implications of Color Vision Research *Journal of the American Optometric Association* June, 1979 50(6):739-43

Peters, George A. A Color-Blindness Test for Use in Vocational Guidance *Personnel and Guidance Journal* May, 1956 pp.572-5

Pickford, R.W. Two Artists With Protan Colour Vision Defects. *British Journal of Psychology* 1965 v.56 4 pp.421-30

Pickford, R.W., Prof. (address by). A Review of Some Problems of Colour Vision and Colour Blindness. *Advancement of Science* Sept.,1958 15-16:104-17

Post, Richard H. Univ. of Mich. Medical School, Ann Arbor, Mich. Colorblindness' Distribution in Britian, France, and Japan: A Review, with Notes on Selection Relaxation. *Eugenics Quarterly* 1963 10:110-18

Post, Richard H. Population Differences in Red and Green Color Vision Deficiency: A Review, and a Query on Selection Relaxation. *Social Biology* 1982 Fal-Win v.29(3-4) pp.299-315

Richards, Oscar W., Ph.D. Limited Improvement of Color Deficient Vision with Colored Filters *Journal of the American Optometric Association* June, 1983 v.54 No.6 pp.537-9

Rosner, Robert S., M.D. Self-Testing Device for Screening Color Vision *American Journal of Ophthalmology* 1962 v.54 p.139

Ruddock, Dr. K.H., Univ. of London 1971 Physics of Colour Vision *Contemporary Physics* v.12 pp.247-56

Rushton, W.A.H. O Say Can You See? *Psychology Today* Oct., 1969 pp.46-53

Rushton, W.A. Visual Pigments and Color Blindness. *Scientific American* March, 1975 pp.64-7

Salvia, John; Ysseldyke, James. Criterion Validity of Four Tests for Red-Green Color Blindness *American Journal of Mental Deficiency* 1972, Jan. v.76:418-22

Sassoon, Humphrey F.; Wise, James B. Diagnosis of Colour-Vision Defects in Very Young Children *Lancet* Feb. 21, 1970 v.1-pt.1:419

Scanlon, James; Roberts, Jean; *Color Vision Deficiencies in Children* U.S. - Data from the National Health Survey, National Center for Health Statistics, Division of Health Examination Statistics. August, 1972

Schmidt, Ingeborg A Sign of Manifest Heterozygosity in Carriers of Color Deficiency *Am. Journal of Optometry and Archives of Am. Academy of Optometry* Aug., 1955 pp.404-408

Shearron, Gilbert F. Color Deficiency and Reading Achievement in Primary School Boys *Reading Teacher* March, 1969 v.22 No.6 pp.510-12,577

Staley, J. J.; Nelson, Willard H.; King, F. J. Color in Discriminative Learning by Children *Journal of Experimental Education* March, 1963 v.31 No.3

Stephenson, Joan. Seeing Yellow *Science Digest* Sept.,1986 p.24

Sutton-Vane, Sybil *Story of Eyes* Viking Press N.Y. c1958

Thompson, Mary A. Color Vision Screening in Prince George's County. *Sight-Saving Review* Winter, 1962 pp.216-7

Thuline, H. C., M.D. Color Blindness in Children: the Importance and Feasibility of Early Recognition *Clinical Pediatrics* May, 1972

Verriest, G. (ed.) Colour Vision Deficiencies VI, Proceedings of the International Symposium, Berlin 1981 *Documenta Ophthalmologica Proceedings* Series 33 c1982 Dr. W. Junk, The Hague

Verriest, G. (ed.) Colour Vision Deficiencies VII, Proceedings of the International Symposium, Geneva 1983 *Documenta Ophthalmological Proceedings* Series 39 c1984 by Martinus Nijhoff/Dr. W. Junk, Pub. The Hague, Boston, Lancaster

Voke, Janet, BSc (Hons), Ph.D., MI Biol. Colour Vision Defects: Their Industrial and Occupational Significance *Nursing Times* Feb.7, 1980 pp.240-43

Voke, Janet. Industrial Requirements and Testing of Colour Vision. *Modern Problems Ophthamological* 1978 19:82-7

Vorster, B.J.; Milner, L. V. Natal Blood Transfusion Service. 2356 Durban 4000, South Africa Colour-Blind Laboratory Technologists (letter) *The Lancet* Dec. 15, 1979

Wedell, Jacelyn; Alden, David G. Color Versus Numeric Coding in a Keeping-Track Task *Journal of Applied Psychology* 1973 v.57-8 No.2 pp.154-9

Weiss, John Deer Do See Color *Outdoor Life* March, 1981 p.64

Welsh, Kenneth W.; Vaughan, John A.; Rasmussen, Paul G. Aeromedical Implications of the X-Chrom Lens For Improving Color Vision Deficiencies *Aviation, Space and Environmental Medicine* March, 1979 50 (3):249-55

Williams, Hugh. Congenital Color Blindness and Its Detection in Children. *Developmental Medicine and Child Neurology* April, 1975 pp.247-51

Wright, William David. *The Rays Are Not Coloured.* Chap. 5, The Unsolved Problem of Daltonism. Hilger. London c1967 pp.67-87

Zeltzer, H.I., O.D. Color Deficiency: Is It Still a Handicap? *Journal of the American Optometric Assoc.* June, 1979 50(6):739-43

Other Persons, Agencies and Companies Concerned with Color Vision Problems:

Federal Highway Administration, U.S. Dept. of Transportation, 400 Seventh St. S.W., Washington, D.C. 20590

Gillilan, Roderick W., O.D., Family Vision Center, 1471 Pearl St., Eugene, OR 97401

Lakeshore Curriculum Materials Co., P.O. Box 6261, 2695 E. Dominguez St. , Carson, CA 90749

March of Dimes Birth Defects Foundation, 1275 Mamaroneck Ave., White Plains, N.Y. 10605

Psychological Corporation, 1250 Sixth Ave., San Diego, CA 92101

X-Chrom Division, Young Contact Lens Laboratories, Inc., 1050 Commonwealth Ave. Boston MA 02215

List of some of the firms that manufacture traffic signals:

(From the Federal Highway Admin. U.S. Dept. of Transportation)

Eagle Signal Controls, 8004 Cameron Road, Austin, Texas 78753 (512) 837-8320

Econolite Control Products, Inc., 3360 East LaPalma, P.O. Box 6150, Anaheim, California 92806 (714) 630-3700

Grammatronix, Inc., 6279 Shier Rings Road, Dublin, Ohio 43017 (614) 889-2511

Safetran Traffic Systems, 1485 Garden of Geds Road, P.O. Box 7009, Colorado Springs, Colorado 80907 (303) 599-5600

3M Company, Safety & Security Systems Division, 3M Center 223 - 3N, St. Paul, Minnesota 55144 (612) 733-4036

Traffic Control Tech., P.O. Box 0399, Liverpool, New York 13088-0399 (315) 451-9500

INDEX

Adams, Anthony J. .... pp.12,19,25,29.

American Optometric Association pamphlet. .... p.24.

Anomaloscopes. .... p.23.

Anomalous trichromats. pp.23,30.

Aqueous humor. .... p.32.

Artists. .... pp.4,13.

Basford, Adelphis Meyer. pp.10,11.

Begbie, G. Hugh. .... p.33.

Bernell Corporation. .... p.26.

Bradshaw, Larry L. .... p.25.

Burnham, Robert W., Hanes, Randall M.,
    Bartleson, D. James. .... pp.1,21.

Clothing. .... pp.5,6.

Cobb, Stephen R. .... p.10.

Collier's Encyclopedia. .... p.33.

Computer Color Vision Test. .... p.25.

Cones. .... p.37.

Cornea. .... p.32.

Cox, Brian J. .... p.25.

Crosby, Bing. .... p.7.

Cruz-Coke, Ricardo. .... pp.4,19,31,32.

Cuisenaire Rods. .... p.9.

Cyan (greensih). .... p.36.

Dalton, John. .... p.33.

Davids, Richard C. .... p.5.

Davidson and Hemmendinger Color Rule. .... p.24.

Deuteranomalous. .... pp.18,23,24.

Deuteranopes. .... pp.18.24,34.

Dichromats. .... pp.18,30.

Dreyer, V. .... p.25.

Dvorine Color Vision Test. .... pp.24,26,27.

Dvorine, Israel. .... pp.9,29.

Edge, Ronald D. (1984). .... p.23.

54

Elks Lodge. ....p.15.
Employment list. ....p.5.
Espinda, Stanley E. ....p.10.

EYE

    Aqueous humor. ....p.32.
    Cones. ....p.37.
    Cornea. ....p.32.
    Iris. ....p.32.
    Lens. ....p.32.
    Optic nerve. ....pp.32,33.
    Pupil. ....p.32.
    Retina. ....pp.32,33.
    Rods. ....p.34.
    Sclera. ....p.32.

Farnsworth D-15 Test. ....pp.24,25,26,27.
Farnsworth, Dean. ....pp.24,25.
Farnsworth Munsell 100 Hue Test. ....p.25.
Federal Highway Admin. Reg. 1980. ....p.4.
Fletcher-Hamblin Simplified Colour Vision Test. ....p.26.
Fletcher, R. ....p.26.
Freese, Arthur S. ....pp.19,32,33.
Functional Color Components (FCC) ....p.9.
Games. ....p.11.

GENETIC COUNSELING

    Genetic Counseling. ....pp.17,19.
    March of Dimes Birth Defects Foundation. ....pp.17,20.
    International Directory of Genetic Services. ....p.20.
    National Association of Vision Program Consultants .p.12.
    National Society for the Prevention of Blindness. ....p.33.

Genetic Counseling. ....pp.17,19.
Genetic Counseling, March of Dimes
    Birth Defects Foundation. ....pp.17,20.
Gillilan, Roderic W. ....p.26.
Goldsmith, Timothy H. ....p.14.
Goldstein, A. G., Borreson, C. R. ....p.30.
Gregory, Richard Langton. ....pp.29,33.
Hailstones and Halibut Bones. ....p.14.
Hammond, Winifred. ....p.33.

Heath, Gordon G. (1963). .... p.17,24,26.
Heath, Gordon G. (1974). .... pp.3,4,10,35.
Hering, Karl. .... p.34.
Heterozygous. .... pp.17,18.
Holmgren Yarn Test. .... pp.24,26.
Homozygous. .... pp.17,18.
Ichikawa Igaku-Shoin Color Vision Test. .... p.27.
Institute of Transportation Engineers. .... p.6.
International Commission on
    Illumination at Cambridge. .... p.6.
International Directory of Genetic Services. .... p.20.
Iris. .... p.32.
Ishihara Color Vision Test. .... pp.24,25,26,27,36.
Johnson, Martin. p.5.
Jonas, Doris and Jonas, David. .... p.14.
Judd, Deane B., Wyszecki, Gunter (1963). .... pp.19,35.
Judd, Deane B., Wyszecki, Gunter (1975). .... p.33.
Kalmus, H. .... pp.18,30.
Kernell, D. .... p.36.
Kessler, Julius. .... p.35.
Kinney, JoAnn S. .... p.29.
Lakeshore Curriculum Materials. .... p.9.
Lampe, John M., Doster, Mildred E.,
    Beal, Barry E. .... p.12.
Land, Edwin. .... p.34.
Learning Disabled children. .... pp.11,12.
Lemonick, Michael. .... p.29.
Lens. .... p.32.
Lincoln, Abraham. .... p.7.
Lions Club. .... p.15.
Litton, Freddie W. .... pp.9,10.
Lyle, W. M. (Jan.,1974). .... p.19.
Lyle, W. M. (Feb.,1974). .... p.19.
Magenta (reddish). .... p.36.
Mantz, Genelle Keithly. .... p.35.
March of Dimes Birth Defects Foundation. .... pp.17,20.
Math Their Way. .... p.9.
Maxwell, J. C. .... p.36.
Mueller, Conrad., Rudolph, Mae. .... p.34.

56

Nagel anomaloscope. ....p.23.

Nagy, Allen L., MacLeod, Donald I. A.,
    Heyneman, Nicholas E., Eisner, Alvin. ....p.18.

National Association of School Nurses. ....p.12.

National Association of Vision Program Consultants........p.12.

National Society for the Prevention of Blindness. ....p.33.

New Spectrum Color Test. ....p.26.

Newman, Paul. ....p.7.

O'Neill, Mary. ....p.4.

Optic nerve. ....pp.32,33.

ORGANIZATIONS

    American Optometric Association pamphlet. ....p.24.

    Elks Lodge. ....p.15.

    International Commission on
    Illumination at Cambridge. ....p.6.

    Lions Club. ....p.15.

    March of Dimes Birth Defects Foundation. ....pp.17,20.

    National Association of School Nurses. ....p.12.

    National Association of Vision Program Consultants...p.12.

    National Society for the Prevention of Blindness. ......p.33.

    P.T.A. ....pp.14,15.

    U.S. Dept. of Health, Education and Welfare. ....p.19.

P.T.A. ....pp.14,15.

Patterson, Elizabeth E. ....p.33.

Paulson, Helen M. ....pp.35,36.

Peters, George. A. .... p.5.

Pickford, R. W. (1964). ....p.4.

Primary colors of light. ....p.23.

Protanomalous. ....pp.18,23.

Protanopes. ....pp.18,24,30,34.

Pseudoisochromatic plates. ....pp.24,26.

Psychological Corporation. .... p.51.

Pulfrich Effect (or Phenomenon). ....p.36.

Pupil. ....p.32.

Reading skills of the color deficient. ....p.12.

Reinfeld, Fred. ....p.26.

Renaldo, John M. ....p.23.

Retina. ....pp.32,33.

Retinex Theory of Color Vision. .... p.34.

Richards, Oscar. Part I. .... p.25.

Richards, Oscar. Part II. .... p.25.

Richer, Stuart., Adams. Anthony J., (April, 1984). .... p.37.

Rods. .... p.34.

Rosenberg, Shirley Sirota. .... pp.11,15,30.

Ruch, F. L. .... p.35.

Sassenroth, Julius M., Pierce, Lajla D.,
    Maddux, Robert E. .... p.9.

Schlanger, Jay L. .... pp.36,37.

Schmidt, Ingeborg (1976).. pp.29,36.

Sclera. .... p.32.

Setright, L.J.K. .... p.30.

Sewell, Julia H. .... PP.9,11.

Sharp, Evelyn. .... p.9.

Shearron, Gilbert F.,Jr. (1964). .... p.12.

Shearron, Gilbert F. .... p.10.

Shute, Donald T., Oshinskie, Leonard. .... p.19.

Siegel, Irwin M. .... pp.35,36.

Snyder, C. R. .... pp.4,10,12.

Stone, Irving. .... p.6.

Structural Arithmetic Blocks (Stern). .... p.9.

TESTS

Anomaloscopes. .... p.23.

Computer Color Visi .... on Test. p.25.

Davidson and Hemmendinger Color Rule. .... p.24.

Dvorine Color Vision Test. .... pp.24,26,27.

Farnsworth D-15 Test. .... pp.24,25,26,27.

Farnsworth Munsell 100 Hue Test. .... p.25.

Fletcher-Hamblin Simplified Colour Vision Test. .... p.26.

Holmgren Yarn Test. .... pp.24,26.

Ichikawa Igaku-Shoin Color Vision Test. .... p.27.

Ishihara Color Vision Test. .... pp.24,25,26,27,36.

Nagel anomaloscope. .... p.23.

New Spectrum Color Test. .... p.26.

Pseudoisochromatic plates. .... pp.24,26.

Thuline, H. C. .... pp.10.18.

Traffic Engineering Division, Eugene, OR .... p.30.

58

Traffic lights. ....pp.6,15,30.
Trichromats. ....pp.18,23.
Tritanomalous. ....pp.18,24.
Tritanopes. ....pp.18,24,34.
U.S. Armed Services. ....p.4.
U.S. Code, 1976 Ed.,v.11, Title 46. ....p.4.
U.S. Dept. of Health, Education and Welfare. ....p.19.
U.S. Dept. of Transportation, Federal Hwy. Admin. ....pp.4,6.
Vehicle Traffic Control Signal Heads, A Standard of
    the Institute of Transportation Engineers. ....p.6.
Vision Screening Guidelines for School Nurses. ....pp.12,13.
Vitreous humor. ....p.32.
Volpe, E. Peter. ....p.18.
Von Helmholtz, Herman. ....p.34.
Waddington, Mary. ....pp.10,12.
Walls, Gordon L., Mathews, Ravenna W. ....p.18.
Water pilots. ....p.4.
Webster's Third New International Dictionary. ....p.33.
Wildman, Peggy Riggs. ....p.9.
Willis, Judith. ....p.17.
Wilson, J. A., Robinson, J. O. ....pp.29,36.
Wright, W. D. ....p.30.
X-Chrom Lens: Case Reports. ....p.36.
X-Chrom Manual. ....p.17.
X-Chromosome. ....pp.17,19.
X-linked ressive traits. .... p.17.
Y-Chromosome. ....p.17.
Young-Helmholtz theory. ....p.34.
Young, Thomas. ....p.34.
Zaba, Joel N. ....p.12.
Zeltzer, H. I. ....pp.29,36.

GLOSSARY

ALLELE — either of a pair of Mendelian characters (as smooth or wrinkled seed in the pea).

ALLELOMORPH — either of a pair of alternative, contrasting, Mendelian characters (as roughness or smoothmess of coats in guinea pigs).

ANOMALOSCOPE — the most precise diagnostic tool for detecting and typing defective color vision. It uses red, green and yellow light sources. The red and green lights may be mixed in various proportions to match the yellow light. Normals make a standard matdh, the color deficient make other matches.

ANOMALOUS — deviating from a general rule, any hereditary peculiarity.

ANOMALOUS TRICHROMAT — a slight defect of color vision in which the proportions of the three primary colors of light required in color mixtures deviate from the normal.

APERTURE — the opening area.

AQUEOUS HUMOR — a limpid fluid occupying the space between the crystalline lens and cornea of the eye.

BASOPHILIC — staining readily with basic stains.

BLIND SPOT — the point in the retina of the eye not sensitive to light where the optic nerve passes through the inner coat of the eyeball.

CHROMATID — one of the paired complex constituent strands of a chromosome.

CHROMOSOME — one of the more or less rodlike chromatin—containing basophilic bodies constituting the genome and chiefly detectable in the mitotic or meiotic nucleus that are regarded as the seat of the genes, consist of one or more intimately associated chromatids functioning as a unit, and are relatively constant in number in the cells of any one kind of plant or animal.

CONTRACTILE — shortening and thickening of a muscle fiber, as in the iris, enabling it to open wider or to narrow the opening.

CORNEA — the transparent part of the coat of the eyeball which covers the iris and pupil and admits light to the interior.

CYAN — a greenish color.

DICHROMAT — one that requires only two primary colors to be mixed in order to match the color spectrum as he sees it.

DEUTERANOMALY — trichromatism in which an abnormally large proportion of green is required to match the spectrum.

ELECTROMAGNETIC (ENERGY) SPECTRUM — energy wavelengths, from a fraction of a centimeter to many thousands of meters.

FOVEA — small pit or depression in the center of the retina, a small rodless area of the retina offering acute vision.

GAMETE — a matured sex or germ cell which is capable of uniting with another of like origin to form a new individual.

GENE — any of the elements in a chromosome by which hereditary characters are transmitted.

GENOME — one haploid set of chromosomes with the genes they contain.

HAPLOID — having the gametic number of chromosomes of half the number characteristic of the somatic cells.

HETEROZYGOUS — possessing genes for both members of at least one pair of allelomorphic Mendelian characters; producing two types of gametes with respect to such a character or characters.

HOMOZYGOUS — dominant for an inheritance factor....possessing genes for only one member of at least one pair of allelomorphic Mendelian characters, producing only one type of gamete with respect to such a character or characters.

HUE — the attribute of colors that permits them to be classed as red, yellow, green, blue or intermediate between any contiguous pair of these.

IRIS — the opaque, muscular curtain or diaphram suspended in the aqueous humor in front of the lens of the eye.

MAGENTA — reddish color.

MEIOTIC — lowering or diminishing.

MENDELIAN — (Mendel, Gregor J.). Mendel's law, the law observed in the inheritance of many characters in animals and plants. In breeding experiments with peas, he showed that the height, color and other characters depend on the presence of determining factors (genes).

MITOTIC — mitosis — cell division in which complex nuclear division usually involving differentiation and halving of chromosomes — indirect cell division.

MONOCHROMAT — one unable to perceive colors. Only black, white and shades of grey are perceived.

NUCLEUS — an element of the protoplasm of most plant and animal cells that is regarded as an essential agent in their growth and reproduction and in the transmission of hereditary characters.

OPTIC NERVE — the bundle of nerves from the eye which extend in a cord from the eye to the brain.

PROTOPLASM — essential living matter of all plant and animal cells.

PSEUDOISOCHROMATIC —(false-same color) plates used for testing color vision. The plates have background dots in greys or colors with contrasting numbers, designs or trails in dots to be distinguished from the background.

PULFRICH EFFECT (Phenomenon) — apparent distortion of motion observed at a distance.

PUPIL — the contractile aperture in the iris of the eye.

RETINA — the sensitive membrane at the back of the eye, which receives the image formed by the lens and is the immediate instrument of vision.

SCLERA — a tough, fibrous coat enclosing the outer surface of the eyeball.

SOMATIC — of the body, physical.

TRICHROMAT — one that requires that three primary colors be mixed in order to match the color spectrum as he sees it; one having normal or nearly normal color vision.

TRITANOPIA — blue (violet) - yellow blindness. (red and green can be perceived).

VITREOUS HUMOR — a transparent, jellylike substance contained in the large posterior part of the eyeball.

X-CHROMOSOME — one of the chromosomes which determine whether a fertilized egg develops into a male or a female. A fertilized egg with two X-chromosomes becomes a female; one with the X Y-chromosome combination becomes a male.

Y-CHROMOSOME — one of the chromosomes in the male sperm. An egg with the X Y combination becomes a male.

(Webster's Second and Third International Dictionaries, Webster's New World Dictionary, Blakiston's Illustrated Pocket Medical Dictionary, and research articles.)

— NOTES —

— NOTES —

— NOTES —

— NOTES —

— NOTES —